The Chair and the Valley

PUB. DATE——————— PRICE —————
UNREVISED AND UNPUBLISHED PROOFS.
CONFIDENTIAL. PLEASE DO NOT QUOTE
FOR PUBLICATION UNTIL VERIFIED WITH
THE FINISHED BOOK. THIS COPY IS NOT
FOR DISTRIBUTION TO THE PUBLIC.
——— THE OPEN FIELD/PENGUIN LIFE ———

The
Chair
and the
Valley

A Memoir of Trauma,
Healing, and the Outdoors

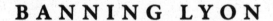

BANNING LYON

THE OPEN FIELD / PENGUIN LIFE

VIKING
An imprint of Penguin Random House LLC
penguinrandomhouse.com

Copyright © 2024 by Banning Lyon

Foreword copyright © 2024 by Jonathan Eig
Penguin Random House supports copyright. Copyright fuels creativity, encourages diverse voices, promotes free speech, and creates a vibrant culture. Thank you for buying an authorized edition of this book and for complying with copyright laws by not reproducing, scanning, or distributing any part of it in any form without permission. You are supporting writers and allowing Penguin Random House to continue to publish books for every reader.

The Open Field/A Penguin Life Book

THE OPEN FIELD is a registered trademark of MOS Enterprises, Inc.

LIBRARY OF CONGRESS CATALOGING-IN-PUBLICATION DATA

[INSERT CIP DATA]

Printed in the United States of America
$PrintCode

Designed by Alexis Farabaugh

Some names and identifying characteristics have been changed to protect the privacy of the individuals involved.

Dear Reader,

Years ago, these words attributed to Rumi found a place in my heart:

> *Out beyond ideas of*
> *wrongdoing and rightdoing,*
> *there is a field. I'll meet you there.*

Ever since, I've cultivated an image of what I call the "Open Field"—a place out beyond fear and shame, beyond judgment, loneliness, and expectation. A place that hosts the reunion of all creation. It's the hope of my soul to find my way there—and whenever I hear an insight or a practice that helps me on the path, I love nothing more than to share it with others.

That's why I've created The Open Field. My hope is to publish books that honor the most unifying truth in human life: We are all seeking the same things. We're all seeking dignity. We're all seeking joy. We're all seeking love and acceptance, seeking to be seen, to be safe. And there is no competition for these things we seek—because they are not material goods; they are spiritual gifts!

We can all give each other these gifts if we share what we know—what has lifted us up and moved us forward. That is our duty to one another—to help each other toward acceptance, toward peace, toward happiness—and my promise to you is that the books published under this imprint will be maps to the Open Field, written by guides who know the path and want to share it.

Each title will offer insights, inspiration, and guidance for moving beyond the fears, the judgments, and the masks we all wear. And when we take off the masks, guess what? We will see that we are the opposite of what we thought—we are each other.

We are all on our way to the Open Field. We are all helping one another along the path. I'll meet you there.

Love,
Maria Shriver

For Jennifer,
and Robert,
and all my friends
from the hospital.

Foreword by Jonathan Eig

In a lawyer's office in Fort Worth, Texas, in the spring of 1993, I met a nervous young man who struggled to make eye contact.

He was pale, slender, and, it seemed to me, achingly sad. He pulled his baseball cap low over his brow, avoiding eye contact. He patted his knee and scratched his nose.

"I wish I could be normal," he said.

I was twenty-eight years old, a newspaper reporter. The young man sitting before me, Banning Lyon, was twenty. Five years earlier, Banning had given his skateboard to a friend. His parents and a guidance counselor had interpreted this is a sign that Banning might be suicidal. Banning tried to tell them that he had bought a new board, that he wasn't depressed or suicidal. It didn't matter. The next day, he was hospitalized, told he would likely stay for two weeks at the Brookhaven Psychiatric Pavilion in Farmers Branch, Texas.

But two weeks became a year, a year in which he endured nightmarish treatment; a year in which his family's insurance company was billed tens of thousands of dollars; a year in which he lost faith in medicine, in his parents, even in himself.

As a local newspaper reporter, I had helped investigate allegations that some private psychiatric hospitals had paid bounties for patients, coerced them into long hospital stays, invented diagnoses, and billed patients' insurance plans until they ran dry. Banning was the first of those patients I met face-to-face.

"They stole a whole year of my life," Banning told me that day in his lawyer's office. "If I live to be eighty-one, then I only lived eighty years."

He reminded me of half my high school friends—awkward, scared, lost, angry. I took an immediate liking to him. But as a newspaper reporter, I was well accustomed to liking people and leaving them behind, writing their stories one day and moving on the next, never learning what would become of them, perhaps even forgetting about them, if truth be told.

It happened by curious chance that at the time I met Banning, a close friend of mine, Bob, a classmate from college, suffered a manic episode and sought inpatient treatment. Like Banning, Bob hoped for a short stint in the hospital but wound up staying much longer. Unlike Banning, however, Bob needed hospitalization, got quality treatment, and seemed to benefit from it. I mention Bob to make sure that anyone reading Banning's book understands that not all inpatient psychiatric care puts profit ahead of patient care. In fact, many doctors complain that America faces a shortage in psychiatric care facilities, especially for teens. According to a recent survey, one third of all high school students report persistent feelings of sadness or hopelessness—an increase of 40 percent from a decade ago.[*] The pandemic has exacerbated many mental health problems,

---

[*] https://www.cdc.gov/healthyyouth/data/yrbs/pdf/YRBS_Data-Summary-Trends_Report 2023_508.pdf.

making access to good care more important than ever. All of this makes a story about bad, predatory care that much more painful, powerful, and worth telling.

Banning and Bob gave me my introduction to mental health treatment. I thought of them recently when I found myself writing about another person who struggled with depressive episodes, a person who twice attempted suicide as a teenager and who voluntarily checked into hospitals numerous times when stress and anxiety became too much for him to bear. His name was Martin Luther King Jr., the subject of my most recent book. King never denied his two adolescent suicide attempts. Years later, when he won the Nobel Peace Prize, the news came to him as he lay in a hospital bed, where, as he told reporters, he had checked in to recover from exhaustion. In the final years of King's life, several friends said he was almost certainly depressed.

Are people with mental health challenges more inclined to be fighters, like Dr. King? Are they made stronger by their ordeals? Are they more apt to become advocates for the rest of us? "You who are in the field of psychology have given us a great word. It is the word maladjusted," King said in 1967 during a speech to the American Psychological Association. King encouraged us to embrace the concept of "creative maladjustment," one that links our internal struggles with the social forces surrounding us, one that helps us in the pursuit of justice, peace, love. There are some things, he said, "to which we should never be adjusted."

When I met him thirty years ago, Banning Lyon seemed like an unlikely candidate to embrace creative maladjustment. Fortunately, he surprised me. It took years, but he found his way, eventually becoming a husband, a father, and a backpacking guide.

It was in his role as a backpacking guide that Banning found his true footing. The outdoors became an antidote, a correction to his year of confinement. On hiking trails, he learned to rely on others and to let others rely on him. Being in nature, with time, with open skies and open minds, led to a powerful revelation: the men and women walking beside him carried psychic burdens of their own. Banning found he could share his story with his fellow backpackers in a way that must have seemed impossible when he tried to share his story with me so many years earlier. "I learned that people weren't stronger or more capable than me," he writes. "They were flawed and broken. They were alcoholics or cutters or parents who'd alienated their kids. And no matter where they'd come from or what they'd survived, we all wanted the same thing: a family where we felt like we belonged."

With growing confidence, Banning opened up about his past. "I began to feel," he writes, "like sharing my story was part of being a guide."

Banning Lyon could be angry now. He was misunderstood and let down by his parents, abused by the medical establishment, and heartbroken by romance, yet the great story he tells is ribboned through with hope and love, without trace of self-pity. In fact, that's what makes Banning a good guide—through this book and, I imagine, through Yosemite National Park or other difficult terrain: he looks for the beauty first, and when he can't see it, he pushes on, with certainty that it lies ahead, somewhere.

Banning's story touches us all, reminding us that mental health is a process, not a destination; it's a walk through the woods, one that might seem painful, even impossible.

"There is no finish line for healing," he writes.

I give thanks that Banning's story didn't end with the article I wrote in 1993. I give thanks for this book, which will stay forever in my mind, where I too can walk on through the difficult terrain, looking ahead toward something beautiful.

—*Jonathan Eig, author of the* New York Times–
bestselling and National Book Award–nominated
biography King: A Life

The
Chair
and the
Valley

Prologue

I was thirty-nine years old when I first saw Yosemite Valley. From the air, its jagged walls and granite spires somehow seemed older than the Earth itself. At one end of the valley stood Half Dome, its iconic summit surrounded by a blanket of snow, like a stone in the middle of a frozen stream. I pressed my face to the window of the plane and gazed at the valley below, the place that would become my home.

The man sitting next to me leaned forward and peered out the window.

"Ever been to Yosemite?" he asked.

"Not yet," I said.

To him, I probably looked like a normal guy, dressed in a pair of jeans and a T-shirt, my knees jammed against the seat in front of me. But I wasn't normal. I was the broken shadow of a person, a fourteen-year-old hiding in an adult's body, still waiting for my parents to pick me up at the airport after they abandoned me. Two years later they would sign me in to a psychiatric hospital operated by a corporation that would eventually plead guilty to the largest health care fraud case in the history of the United States.

The man next to me leaned back in his seat.

"Are you planning on going to the valley soon?"

"I'm flying out for a job interview," I said, "to be a backpacking guide."

His eyes grew wide. "In Yosemite?"

"Yeah, my interview's tomorrow."

I looked back out the window. I didn't like looking at people when I spoke to them. After having been forced to sit in a quiet room and stare at a wall for months at a time, I didn't trust people anymore. I couldn't count how many times I'd listened to my friends shriek and cry for help while the hospital staff held them down and strapped them to their beds. My fiancée had survived that place when she was a teenager too. Until years later, when her heroin addiction killed her, and almost killed me.

I was still staring out the window when the man spoke again.

"I haven't been to Yosemite in years," he said. "I'll never forget the first time I drove into the valley. I remember getting out of my car and thinking it was the first place that ever made me believe in God."

I didn't say anything, I just watched the valley below slowly drift into the distance. Four months later I'd see Yosemite in person—and it wouldn't make me believe in God. For the first time in my life, it would make me believe in myself.

I Don't Want You

The journey that would lead me to become a backpacking guide didn't begin in a psychiatric hospital or Yosemite. It began in a small stucco house in the foothills of Sonoma, California, twenty-six years before, when my parents first sent me away.

I was born in Southern California, the son of a pilot and a travel agent who had gotten married just before the bloodiest years of the Vietnam War. Until I was eleven, my life seemed perfect. Dad took me on weekend trips around North America. We went hiking and sailing and sat under trees and ate lunch together. When he was home, we wandered through the hills near our house, searching under rocks and logs for snakes and lizards. Once, when I caught a five-foot-long gopher snake, Dad said we should take it home and show my mom.

"Look what we found today," he told her, smiling.

I pulled the snake out of a pillowcase and Mom screamed at the top of her lungs. Dad and I burst into laughter. Mom almost passed out.

It wasn't until their bitter divorce and custody battle that Mom finally sent me and my older sister to live in Sonoma with my dad and stepmom, Linda. It was easy to like Linda, with her long blond hair and flight attendant smile, but she was in her late twenties and had never had kids. Even as a thirteen-year-old, I could tell she didn't know how to deal with two teenagers. By the time I'd started seventh grade, my sister Adrienne had gotten her driver's license. I hardly saw her again after that.

A year later, when Adrienne was a senior and ready to go to college, Linda and I began to argue. She'd ask me to do chores and I'd rush through them, only to have her ask me to do more. I'd always been free to do what I wanted before, so I pushed back. Halfway through the summer of 1985, Linda had had enough.

"I think you need to go back and live with your mom," she said. "You'll be happier there. Not to mention, she's always reminding us she still has full custody."

Before Dad married Linda, he was my best friend. We'd talk and laugh and work in the yard together. But after my parents' divorce, he seemed quiet and distant. He spent more time away. And when he was home, we only did things with Linda. He wasn't my dad anymore; he was her husband now. When Linda finally told me I needed to go live with my mom again, he walked out of the room as if he hadn't heard her.

"I don't want to live with Mom," I said, following him. "I want to live with you. I want to go hiking and catch snakes again. I miss you."

"Give her a call anyway, son," he said.

I was heartbroken. My dad was worse than dead; he was gone. I almost began to cry, but I didn't want him to see my tears. He didn't even look at me as he walked away.

I'll never forget watching him as he left that afternoon. I wondered why he had given up on me, why he refused to remember how close we'd been before he married Linda. The moment reminded me of something he once told me when I was younger, after we had stopped during a hike to rest in the shade of a tree. We were drinking water from his old metal canteen when I saw a plane overhead.

"Are you ever afraid of crashing, Dad?" I asked.

He shook his head and grinned, the way he always did when he was certain of something.

"Nope," he said. "Never. It doesn't even occur to me. I always imagine good things happening. There's no point in thinking about what could go wrong."

Since my parents' divorce, maybe that's all I was to my dad, something bad that had happened to him, a reminder of something that had gone wrong. But to me, our memories together were the happiest moments of my life. I couldn't understand why I was only a part of his past and not a part of his future.

I never knew why my parents divorced. My mom said he had cheated on her, but I didn't believe it. I didn't believe anything my mom said. I hardly knew her. I knew her parents had been poor and she grew up in the South, and now she ran a travel agency and she loved her Cadillac and her Rolex. But she didn't feel like my mom. She acted like an android that had been programmed to take care of me, with her short black hair and ice-blue eyes as mysterious as the glaciers I'd seen in Alaska. I knew she loved me, but only under the right conditions.

I called her the next day. She sounded happy to hear from me, although I didn't know why.

"Linda said I need to come live with you," I said.

"Honey, I'd love that, but I don't have room for you. I live in a tiny condo in Newport Beach now. I only have one bedroom. You're thirteen. You need your own room."

"But Linda said I can't stay here," I told her. "She said you have full custody."

Mom didn't say anything. I peered around the corner of the kitchen and saw Linda sitting on the sofa, listening to me. She smiled and gave me a thumbs-up.

"Why don't you talk to Linda?" I said to Mom, tears filling my eyes.

"I don't want to talk to her," she snapped. "Tell them I don't have room for you."

Week after week Linda asked me to try again. I'd stand in the kitchen, tethered to our wall-mounted phone, and dial Mom's number while I leaned against the wall to hide my shame. But no matter how many times I called, nothing ever changed. Linda would tell me to call again, then she'd sit in the living room and eavesdrop after Dad left the room. Mom always said the same thing, like her circuits were broken.

"I don't have room for you, honey."

Finally, weeks later, angry and tired of the phone calls, Mom told me to fly to Dallas to stay with my aunt and uncle until she could join me there. I'd gone to visit them once when I was a child. Other than that one trip, the only thing I remembered about Texas was the blistering summer sun.

It was July when my uncle Dave stood waiting for me at the Dallas airport. He was tall and thin and had deep-set eyes and a solemn voice. We walked in silence together past the magazine stands and restaurants that lined the terminal. Then he patted me on the shoulder as if he were sorry for me, sorry that I didn't have a family. Not because they had been killed but because they didn't want me anymore.

Dallas was hot and humid and filled with houses built in flat rows bordering straight streets, like an enormous suburban waffle iron. Neighbors stood in their yards every evening and watered the grass, their shadowed figures backlit against a huge sunset and open sky. My aunt and uncle and their two daughters agreed to take care of me until Mom could sell her condo and move to Texas. My first week "living under their roof," as my uncle Dave called it, consisted of church four times a week, a blessing before every meal, and a fifteen-minute prayer circle before bed.

The only things that felt familiar were my uncle Dave's keepsakes from Vietnam. He had been a fighter pilot in the navy and flown alongside my dad over cities like Hanoi and Vinh and Thanh Hóa. His study was filled with memorabilia from the war. Every day I would wander to that quiet corner of the house and stare at the black-and-white photographs of him and my dad and the times they had shared. Dad looked so young, standing with his flight helmet under one arm and smiling at me from somewhere off the coast of Vietnam. I remembered the same photograph hanging in Dad's study when I was a little boy, but the image of him seemed different now. I felt like I'd lost him forever. Sometimes I'd take the picture off the wall and sit on the floor and cry while I stared at him and wondered why he had to marry someone who didn't want me.

I started eighth grade that summer, five months before my classmates and I would watch the space shuttle *Challenger* disintegrate on TV. Every weekday morning my older cousins drove me to school, and we'd ignore each other while I sat in the back seat and gazed out the window, at cars filled with smiling families who still had one another. Then I'd come home and do my homework and help my uncle Dave around the house before slinking off to my room. But none of it made any difference. We all knew I wouldn't be staying for long, and that no amount of chores or prayers would ever make us a family.

Mom called every week to check on me. She asked about Adrienne, but I hadn't spoken to her, and my dad and Linda hadn't called me since the day they sent me to Texas. When I turned fourteen that September, I waited by the phone for Dad to call me. He never did. I went to bed in tears.

By Christmas, I'd stopped looking at his picture.

I was doing my homework in my room one evening when Uncle Dave knocked on my door and handed me the phone.

"Hi, honey," Mom said. "I've got some good news. I'm moving to Dallas next month to live with your aunt Martha and uncle John." Martha was Mom's younger sister. "You can move there and live with me. We'll look for an apartment once I'm settled there and find a job."

Uncle Dave drove me and my few belongings over to meet Mom when she arrived a couple of weeks later. We pulled up in front of the house to see her sorting through a pile of clothing in the back seat of her Cadillac. She threw open her arms and I gave her a hug because I didn't want to disappoint her. I hadn't seen her since the day I'd moved to Sonoma, two years before, when I walked into her bedroom to say goodbye. I remembered sitting on the edge of her bed and putting my hand on her shoulder. She didn't say anything. She just lay there like a corpse wrapped in her thin cotton sheets. She used to cry all the time after Dad left. She even stopped talking for a while. As far as I was concerned, my mom had been gone for nearly three years.

Uncle Dave grabbed two bags of clothing out of her car and started for the house. Mom walked around to the trunk and dug through a box.

"Guess what I bought for you," she said, handing me a brand-new skateboard. "I remember how much you loved skating when you were a little boy."

I'd forgotten my old yellow skateboard and our brief love affair. Mom's gift conjured memories of skating barefoot and coasting around the street in front of our driveway. I wanted to be grateful, but it was hard to feel anything other than disappointment about my parents. I gave Mom another hug and began carrying my things inside.

Our room above Aunt Martha and Uncle John's garage was dusty and hot and too small for me and my mom, but my days of church and bedtime prayer circles were over. Mom worked all day and looked for apartments when she wasn't home. Uncle John lounged in his recliner and watched TV while Aunt Martha sat at the kitchen table, rereading her decades-old pile of tabloid magazines. Other than saying "Good morning" or "Good night," they only spoke to me if I was standing in front of their television.

I spent all my free time on my new skateboard, racing around in the Texas heat before retreating to the house, where I'd peel off my shirt, sit in the air-conditioning, and bury my face in the pages of a *Thrasher* skateboarding magazine. The black-and-white newsprint pages were crammed full of articles and pictures and artwork. Advertisements mocked parents. Skaters in wigs posed as worried moms wagging their fingers. There were ads for bands with names like Black Flag, Minor Threat, and Suicidal Tendencies. Every page read like an angry Declaration of Independence.

Month after month I'd kick my skateboard down to the local skate shop and buy the newest issue. I didn't even bother going back home to read them. I'd sit on the sidewalk outside the shop and commit each word and picture to memory, all of them symbols of a world free of my parents and the suffering they had caused me.

"I want you to try to go back to California and live with your dad," Mom said.

It was a weeknight in June, nearly a year since we had moved into the room above Martha and John's garage. I'd been skating out front when Mom got home from work and waved for me to come inside. Those words were the first thing she had said to me all day.

I stopped in the doorway and stared at her. She stood behind a short stack of half-unpacked boxes, still wearing one of the designer suits she always wore to the travel agency where she had gotten a job. I almost shouted at her, but I knew it wouldn't help. After my being shuffled around for the last two years, no one seemed to care what I wanted anyway.

"Try?" I asked. "What do you mean, 'try'?"

"You're always saying how much you miss California," she said, sweetening her voice. "It's summer now. You're out of school. You should call your dad to see if you can visit for a while. Maybe he'll let you stay this time."

I'd gotten used to my mom manipulating me. She'd try to convince me to do something and I'd refuse. Then she'd cry or yell at me, hoping to change my mind. I wondered if she had done the same thing to my dad.

I tossed my skateboard on the bed. "So they don't know I'm coming, and you want me to stay?"

"They owe me child support and alimony, Banning. And now they're building some stupid house." Mom fell silent. She clenched her jaw. "When you go back, I want you to go through their bills and find some credit card receipts and send them to me. I can take those bills to court and get the money we deserve, money to get you clothes for school, maybe even another skateboard."

"What the fuck does it matter, Mom? I'm going to live with them now, right?"

She slammed the door and stormed downstairs. I couldn't help but feel sorry for her. I knew she still loved my dad, even though she said he had cheated on her and then left us for Linda.

I dug the phone out from under a pile of Mom's clothing and stared at it. I hadn't heard my dad's voice in two years. I wanted to hate him instead of missing him so much. I dialed his number and he answered a moment later. "Banning," he said, almost shouting. "How are you, son?" He sounded ecstatic. It was awkward talking to him again, like I was acting in a school talent show. "I was thinking maybe I can come visit," I said. Linda got on the extension, her voice still young and friendly. "We'd love to see you," she said. "We'll call the airport and get a pass for you." They both still worked for Western Airlines. Linda rambled on and on about their new house before they finally hung up.

I slumped against the wall next to my bed. "They never even call to say hi or check on me," I said to my skateboard. "And now they're happy to see me?"

Uncle John dropped me off at the airport later that week. I'd spent countless hours of my childhood walking through airports with my dad.

We'd board the plane before everyone else and I'd sit in the cockpit and he'd introduce me to the crew while they went through the preflight checklist. Sometimes he'd call the tower and let me talk to the air traffic controllers. "My son's gonna be a pilot, just like his dad," he said once. The crew laughed and laughed. Then he put his hat on my head and walked me down the aisle to my seat while he chatted with the passengers. I felt like the luckiest kid in the world.

But now I sat alone in the cabin and flew back to California so I could lie and steal in exchange for what was left of my family. I propped my forehead against the cold plastic window and stared at the world below, wondering if anything I did really mattered anymore.

Dad was standing at the gate when I arrived in San Francisco. He looked happier than the last time I'd seen him, when he dropped me off at the same terminal and said goodbye.

"Hey, son," he said. "How was the flight?"

"Nice. Bad landing though. Two bumps." Critiquing landings for him was an old ritual.

"Check any luggage?"

"Yeah, just one bag," I said. I'd left a lot of stuff behind because I didn't want him to suspect that I planned on staying with them.

"Well, let's stop by baggage claim. Then we'll pick up lunch on the way to the house." He gave my shoulder a squeeze. "Can't wait for you to see it."

He hardly spoke during the drive. Every once in a while I'd look at him and wonder if my dad was still in there somewhere, but he seemed even more distant now. He didn't laugh or joke with me. He didn't talk about the years we had spent together. I felt like a hitchhiker, stuck in a car with a stranger.

We passed through Sonoma an hour later. I hadn't seen the town since I'd moved to Texas, and I'd forgotten how much I missed it, with its red-winged blackbirds and foggy mornings and vineyards planted in neat rows that unfurled across the valley. Dad swung a left at a barely familiar intersection and drove into the hills where we used to go hiking. We came to a narrow road and followed it through the woods before coming to a stop in front of a beautiful new house. It looked just like I had imagined, surrounded by oak and bay trees and wild grass. But there was a not-quite-rightness to everything, as if I were stepping into a life where I didn't belong.

Linda was working in the barn. She came running up the driveway and threw her arms around me. "I'm so glad you came to visit," she said. She hadn't changed at all, with her sunny smile and faded blue jeans, like a cover girl for California. I couldn't help but think of all the times she had told me to go live with my mom.

Dad and I spent the next few days working around the house. We trimmed trees and loaded the bed of the truck with trunks and limbs to take to the dump. Then we'd drive back up the hill and go hiking through the woods before stopping to eat lunch in the shade of a tree.

"I bet there's a lot of snakes around here," I said one afternoon.

He nodded quietly as if he'd never considered it.

"Remember that huge gopher snake I caught? The one we showed Mom."

Dad winced like he had bitten his cheek. The space between us suddenly grew larger. He closed his eyes and took a breath and then packed up what was left of his lunch.

"We should get going," he said, turning for the house. "There's still a lot of work to do."

I felt so stupid. I imagined chasing him and hugging his waist. I wanted to beg him to come back to me, the proud dad who used to introduce me to passengers and let me wear his hat. But he was gone now, and he wasn't coming back.

Mom called a few times that week. She'd chat for a couple of minutes before asking how "things were going," which seemed to be some vague reminder for me to go through Dad's bills. I didn't plan on stealing anything for her, but concealing her plot made me feel dishonest. And although I wasn't sure if Dad and Linda would let me stay, I knew if they found out what Mom had asked me to do they'd put me on the next plane back to Texas.

Later that week the three of us sat around the kitchen table and talked over dessert. The moment we finished our ice cream, I jumped to my feet and started carrying the dishes to the kitchen. I knew I needed to impress them if I wanted to stay. Dad walked over from the table while I was filling the sink with water.

"Sit back down, son," he said. "Linda and I need to talk to you. We'll do the dishes later."

My heart sank. I followed them into the living room and slouched in one of the chairs.

"We love having you here," Linda told me, "and it's obvious you're doing your best to be good, but . . ." She looked at Dad as if she needed help. He was staring out the window. "You can't live here, Banning," she said. "Your mother still has full custody. You're only fourteen."

I looked away. I couldn't understand why they didn't want me. I almost told Linda that my mom didn't want me either, but I knew it wouldn't matter. Dad stood and walked to the kitchen and began washing the dishes. He wouldn't look at us. I wondered what I'd done to make them not love me. Linda kept talking while I watched him. Her words sounded muted and distant.

Dad took me to the airport later that week. We drove with the windows down. The air was cool and smelled of eucalyptus trees. I remember gazing at the blue civic center as we passed through Marin. It seemed sad to waste such a beautiful day.

We stopped at the terminal and I felt Dad give me a hug. "I love you, son," he said. He helped me check my bag at the curb, then pulled out his wallet and handed me a dollar.

"Make sure to call your mom when you arrive."

I landed in Dallas hours later. I found a pay phone and dialed my aunt and uncle's number.

"Valerie!" Aunt Martha shouted. "Your son's on the phone!"

Mom picked up the other line.

"Hey, Mom. I'm at DFW. Dad told me to call you."

"What happened?" she asked.

"They sent me back." I leaned my forehead against the wall next to the phone and closed my eyes. "I need you to come get me."

"I told you he would screw this up," Martha said. "You're just like your miserable father, Banning. I hope you don't cheat on your wife and break up *your* family." She slammed down the receiver.

Mom was quiet for a long time before she spoke. "You call your dad and Linda, and you tell them to get you a flight back to California. Do *not* come back here. I don't want you."

Then she hung up.

I stared at the polished chrome of the pay phone and listened to the dial tone. My distorted reflection gazed back at me.

"What did I do wrong?" I said. "Why does this keep happening?"

I used the rest of my quarters to call three more times, but Mom or Martha kept hanging up on me. I checked all the other pay phones, poking my finger into the coin return in search of a quarter. I never found one.

The terminal was quiet and empty. I sat at a nearby gate and listened to the distant murmur of voices and people. Then I picked up my bag and started walking. I didn't know where to go. I stopped near baggage claim and gazed out the windows at a street spotted with the oil of a million cars. The automatic doors slid open and the humid Texas air swallowed me. I stepped outside and stood alone in the heat. The wavering buzz of cicadas filled the air.

"I guess no one's coming to get me," I said to them.

I wandered back inside and sat in a row of black plastic chairs that faced a large window and looked out onto the airfield. Each of the chairs had a small coin-operated television mounted to the end of one arm. The seats were hard and uncomfortable. Outside, planes departed and arrived. The muted growl of their engines rumbled through the glass. I'd always loved that sound. I sat and watched the planes for a long time.

I turned to my little red bag and laid my hand on its side.

Everything I have is in the chair next to me, I thought. *I don't have a family anymore. I'm alone now.*

After several hours and two collect calls to Martha and John's house, I went to baggage claim to get my other bag and then called the operator. She connected me to what sounded like the police. A man with a thick Texas accent answered the phone. I told him I was stuck at the airport, and he asked for my name and age. I said I was fourteen.

"Where are your parents?" he asked.

I almost started crying. I didn't know how to answer the question. There was too much to explain.

"My dad's back in California," I said. "My mom was supposed to pick me up."

"She might be held up in traffic. It's still rush hour."

A flight attendant standing nearby looked at me. I hid between the partitions that separated the phones and lowered my voice.

"She's still at home," I said. "She keeps hanging up on me."

The officer was quiet for a moment. His voice was low and calm when he spoke again.

"Don't you worry, son. This is probably just some misunderstanding. What's her number?"

I gave him Aunt Martha's phone number. Then he asked for the number printed on the pay phone. I read it to him and he told me to stay put until he called back. The phone rang a few minutes later.

"Your mother's on her way," he said. "She'll be there in an hour or so. If she's not, you call me back, son. Understand?"

An hour later my uncle John's huge brown Cadillac pulled up outside the terminal. John sat expressionless behind the wheel. Aunt Martha was in the passenger seat next to him. Mom sat in back. She had been crying. She and Martha looked furious, both of them glaring at me while John stared out the windshield. I thought about running away, but I had nowhere to go. I put my bags in the trunk and then got in the car. Mom started yelling at me. "Why did you have to come back?" she shouted. Aunt Martha turned around and joined her. They both looked hysterical. Mom crying and screaming. Martha's eyes wide and hateful. Mom slapped me once, hard. Then again. And again. Quick, sharp slaps. I covered my face and turned away. She slapped the back of my head. I heard myself crying. I begged her to stop. Mom had never hit me before. She sounded like she had lost her mind, screaming and wailing in rage and grief. By the time we were on the highway, she was crying too hard to hit me anymore.

"I'm sorry, Mom," I cried. "I'm sorry." I kept saying it. I don't know why.

Mom finally fell quiet and stared out the window. Aunt Martha didn't speak either.

Uncle John never said a word.

2

Suicidal Tendencies

A few months after Mom left me at the airport, we moved out of Martha and John's house into a two-bedroom apartment down the street. She never apologized for hitting me, and I never asked about it. I got a job bagging groceries at a nearby store. A month later I started ninth grade. The rest of my time was committed to skateboarding and punk rock and the ever-growing notion that the only person I could trust was me.

Mom suffered from depression. I knew it as a child. She worked all the time and slept a lot and her smile looked like something she'd rehearsed in the mirror. She bought nice things to make herself happy, like her 1979 Cadillac Seville, the same color as her frosty blue eyes. When I was a kid, she used to make my sister Adrienne practice piano every day. She insisted on cutting my hair until I was eleven. She made sure Adrienne got straight As. We weren't kids; we were symbols of the happiness Mom had always wanted for herself.

Shortly after the divorce, she started waking us in the middle of the night. We'd sit at the kitchen table in the dark and cry while she talked about how lonely she was without Dad. "We're all alone," she would say. "You're the man of the house now." It was a nightly ritual. Adrienne was a teenager back then and finally stopped coming out of her room, so Mom would get me out of bed and we would sit in the dark while I stared at the floor and listened to her rant about my unfaithful dad and his terrible girlfriend, Linda. That's probably why Adrienne never called her. She'd gone to college and never looked back.

Four years later, living in Dallas, Mom had hardly changed. The only difference was her silence. She didn't talk about my dad anymore, or how much I looked like him, or that she had finally accepted being stuck with me. Instead, she carried those unspoken words in her body as if she had swallowed something that was slowly poisoning her. Every evening she'd come home and shuffle into the kitchen like an overworked farm horse, tired and bent from years of work and loneliness. Then she'd microwave a frozen dinner and wander off to her room and stare at her television. I hated seeing her like that. I loved my mom. She wasn't a monster. She was just sad and lonely like me.

But life with my mom wasn't always terrible. We had good days too. We went out to eat sometimes and she'd tell stories about happier days ahead, how she planned to save money and buy a real house. "Maybe we'll even move back to California someday," she'd say. I didn't believe it. But listening to her daydream about a happier life was better than watching her come home and eat dinner alone in her room.

Life in Dallas improved too. I made friends at work and school, and skateboarding helped me build a small community. The moment I saw another person on a skateboard, I knew I had made a friend. And not just because we shared a common love for skating or learning tricks, but also because we loved the culture and the music. We read the same magazines. We listened to the same bands. We were a family.

Within months I felt like I had shed my skin and become someone else, someone unique and confident. I liked who I was now. And for the first time, girls liked me too. My first girlfriend was a black-haired goth girl covered in freckles who had transferred to our school in the middle of the year. The first time she walked into the cafeteria, the whole room fell silent. She stood in the middle of the entrance, wearing a long white dress trimmed with lace. She was the prettiest girl in school. The second she saw me, she walked across the cafeteria and said hi. I almost dropped my tray. I had never felt so special. Sometimes she would come over before my mom got home from work, and we would curl up on my bed and listen to music, and I would kiss the back of her neck while she gently grazed her nails up and down my arms. My life wasn't perfect. I still missed California. But settling in Dallas was better than being bounced from house to house like an unwanted package.

Mom and I had lived in the apartment for nearly four months when she came home from work one afternoon and asked for help with the groceries. I grabbed a few bags and carried them into the apartment. Mom walked in a moment later.

"I found you a therapist today," she said.

I spun around and stared at her. "Why?"

"I thought it would be a good idea," she said. "I know you're not happy here."

"Then get yourself a therapist. You need one more than I do."

"I already made an appointment," she said, walking away. "For *you*. And you're going."

I met my therapist a week later. Sam was tall and lanky and maybe fifty years old. He had snowy white hair and keen blue eyes. He wore a shiny gray polyester suit and a bolo and a pair of cowboy boots. He reminded me of my uncle John's favorite Texasism, "He's all hat and no horse."

"Your mom tells me you like music," Sam said, closing the door to leave her waiting in the lobby.

"Yeah. I do, but she hates it."

"Why do you say that?"

"Because she says so all the time."

He smiled and sat in the chair opposite me. "Do you get along with your mom?"

I thought of her leaving me at the airport and then slapping me while I cowered in the back seat of the car, but I didn't want her to get in trouble.

"I guess," I said with a shrug. "She works a lot. We don't see each other much."

"And your folks are divorced?"

"Yeah. My dad and stepmom still live in California. He's a pilot."

"Do you miss him?" Sam asked.

I nodded. I didn't like admitting it.

"Your mom says you miss California."

"Yeah," I said. "I don't really like Texas."

"Why not?"

"The weather sucks. The food's good, though."

Sam cracked a grin and leaned back in his seat and propped his foot on his knee. I'd never been to a therapist, but he wasn't what I'd expected. He didn't take notes or ask stupid questions. There was kindness in his voice.

"So tell me about your favorite music," he said. "What's on your turntable right now?"

"*My War* by Black Flag. I listen to it every day. That and Minor Threat." I tipped my chair back to see if he'd correct me. He didn't.

"What do you like about Black Flag?"

"Their songs are about being depressed and angry," I said. "You can hear it in their music."

My mom had never asked a single meaningful question about my music; all she did was complain about it. But Sam seemed to genuinely care. Week after week Mom would drive me to my appointment and I'd share a favorite song or album with him, and we'd talk about what they meant to me. It didn't feel like therapy; it felt more like a friendship. He didn't complain about my clothing or spiked hair. He didn't yell at me for playing my music too loud. He asked about my feelings. He was the first adult I'd trusted in a long time, and he earned that trust without my realizing it. I probably wouldn't have admitted it to anyone, but I loved Sam for caring about me.

It was January of 1987 when my friend Jack broke the deck of his skateboard. I had saved some money from my job at the grocery store to buy a new deck, so I offered to give him my old one. We walked to the shop after school, got my new board, and spent the rest of the afternoon skating before heading home after dark.

The next morning, a group of friends were standing in the hallway at school. "I heard you gave your board away," one of them asked. I told them Jack had broken his old deck and that I'd given him mine.

"Check it out," I said, pulling the board out of my locker. "Brand-new mini Caballero."

The bell rang and we walked to class. As the day went on, at least three or four other people asked why I had given away my board, and with each repetition the question sounded more serious. By the time I walked out of my last period, I began to wonder if I had done something wrong.

I left school that afternoon and skated toward home. I was waiting to cross the street when a small red car pulled up. A woman leaned over from the driver's seat and rolled down the passenger window. It was my school counselor.

"I've been looking for you," she said. "I want to talk to you about your skateboard."

She had the same annoying look of concern on her face as everyone else who had come looking for me that day. For a moment I considered telling her the whole story and showing her my new board, but no one ever seemed to listen to me, so I skated off after mumbling something about needing to get home. As soon as I rounded the corner of our apartment building, I saw Mom's car parked out front.

I stared at our apartment for a long time, wondering why she had come home. She never left work early, and the sight of her car in her parking spot made my stomach turn. I walked to the door and eased my key into the lock. Mom ran out of her bedroom the moment she heard me.

"Your counselor called me at work today," she said. "She told me you gave away your skateboard and you're planning on killing yourself."

"What? No!"

"Then why'd you tell a friend of yours that everyone would be happier without you around?"

I couldn't count how many times I'd said the same thing to my friends. Half of them felt the same way about their parents. I had even said it to my mom before, but now she suddenly seemed to care.

"Probably because you tried to ship me back to California and didn't pick me up at the fucking airport."

"So you really said that?" she asked.

"I don't know. Why are you so surprised? I've said that to *you*."

Mom sat on the arm of the sofa. She took a deep breath and pressed her palms to her eyes. "Well, I made an appointment to see Sam tonight, and he's going out of his way to meet us."

"Tonight? Why? We were just there a few days ago."

"Honey, I'm not mad at you. I'm scared."

I had grown so used to my mom's complaining that her suddenly worrying about me seemed strange. I regretted upsetting her. I turned for my bedroom and grabbed my new board.

"I never should've given away my fucking skateboard," I said.

Mom and I arrived at Sam's office a few hours later. It was strange to see the building at night, with its empty parking lot and green fluorescent lights. I wondered if there was some way to convince Sam this was all a misunderstanding.

"So your mom tells me you gave away your skateboard," he said when we were alone in his office.

"Yeah, and I bought a new one. My friend Jack broke his, so I gave him my old board."

Sam narrowed his eyes as if he were trying to read my mind. "Have you been depressed lately?"

I almost laughed. He asked the question like he hadn't even heard me. Every adult who had asked why I'd given away my skateboard seemed to ignore the fact that I'd given it to my best friend and bought a new one.

I deflated in my chair and sighed. "I don't know."

"Have you thought about hurting yourself?"

The question sounded weird. I shook my head.

"Did you tell a friend of yours that everyone would be better off without you around?"

"Yeah," I said. "I've said that to my mom for months, ever since she tried to pawn me off on my dad."

"Have you considered suicide?"

"Sam, I bought a new skateboard. Why would I buy a new board if I wanted to kill myself?"

"That's what we're trying to understand, Banning."

Sam stood and retrieved two sheets of paper from his desk and handed them to me. They were photocopies of drawings I had made in the margins of my school notes. One of them was a portrait of a horned and bearded face that looked vaguely satanic. The other was a drawing of a boxing glove holding a knife. A creepy smiling face peered out from behind it.

"Are these your drawings?" he asked.

"Well, yeah. Kind of."

"Kind of?"

"They're from two of my favorite Black Flag albums," I said. "I've read you lyrics from them. I copied them. They aren't *mine*."

"Then why did you write 'Suicidal Tendencies' in one of your books?"

I started laughing. He raised his eyebrows.

"They're a band, Sam."

We spoke for half an hour before he asked to talk to my mom alone. She touched my arm as I left the room. The door opened two minutes later.

"I'd like to see you both again tomorrow afternoon," he said.

Mom hardly spoke during the drive home. She stared over the hood of the car in silence, gazing through the traffic at something far away. I began to wonder if I had made a terrible mistake by giving away my skateboard, and if whatever I had set into motion was out of my control now.

Mom picked me up from school the next day and drove me to Sam's office. We walked into the lobby and she sat with her hands folded in her lap while I paced around the room. Everything felt wrong. I never saw Sam twice in a week and Mom never left work to take care of me. Even her expression seemed different, like a kid sitting in a principal's office, staring at her knees.

I could hear two men speaking on the other side of the wall. One of them was Sam, his voice pitched high as he wrapped up the conversation. The other voice made me sick and scared. I recognized it before the door opened.

Dad and I still looked the same. Both of us tall and thin. He grinned as if we had bumped into each other in the grocery store. I wanted to curl up in a ball and disappear.

"Hi, son," he said. "Sam and I have been talking. Sounds like a lot's going on."

I shrugged and looked at the floor.

"Let's all sit down," Sam said, gesturing into his office.

Mom slouched in the chair next to me. Dad sat in another a few feet behind her. They were both so consumed with ignoring each other that it was difficult to notice anything else.

"Banning, your parents and I have been talking, and we believe it would be in your best interest if you were hospitalized."

I almost jumped out of my chair. "What? Why?"

"We're concerned for your safety," he said. "It's only for two weeks."

"Two weeks? But what about school?"

"They're fine with you being gone for a short time," Mom said. "You can make up your schoolwork when you get back, just like being sick."

"Sick! For two weeks!" A sudden urge to run rushed through me. "I don't want to go."

"Honey, you have to . . ."

Sam interrupted her. "Banning, I want you to trust me. Please. It's only a two-week evaluation. No one wants to force you to go."

Force? What the fuck does that mean?

Sam asked me to leave the room for a few minutes. I sat alone in the lobby and imagined running out the door, but I had no idea where to go. I finally decided that bad food and nurses in white were probably better than juvenile detention.

Mom stepped out of Sam's office and closed the door.

"I don't want to go," I said.

"It's just for two weeks, honey. I've already packed your bags."

Sam reappeared a moment later. Dad stood behind him.

"Can I call my friends before I go?" I asked Sam.

"You'll have a chance to do that later," he said.

Mom drove us to the hospital and then walked inside. Dad and I stood in the parking lot and talked while I leaned against a car parked next to his rental. "I'm not suicidal," I told him. "I just gave away my skateboard, but I bought a new one."

"I have to trust Sam, son. We're concerned about you. It's only for two weeks."

I stopped listening and stared into the distance. The January sky was dark blue and the last of the day's light was nothing but a glowing sapphire line on the horizon. A row of grackles were perched on a telephone line on the far side of the parking lot, calling to one another. I turned and glanced at the hospital. It looked like a prison. Thick metal screens covered all the windows.

Dad followed me inside and we stepped into a small office. The woman working in admissions moved a stack of papers around the desk and asked Sam and my parents for their signatures and initials. I stood toward the back of the room. No one spoke to me. Mom touched my shoulder once. We left the office and I felt Dad give me a hug. "Take care, son," he said. He stayed behind as Sam followed me and Mom to a pair of double doors. A staff member pulled a set of keys on a retractable wire from their belt and stuck one of them in a metal panel on the wall. There was a faint hum and a click as the doors unlocked.

Sam and the staff member followed me and my mom into a space the size of a large elevator. There was another pair of doors in front of us, each of them fitted with a narrow wire-reinforced security window. I could see people inside sitting at tables. The doors behind us closed and then a lock clicked and the ones in front of us opened.

The four of us stepped into a large foyer. A sickening cloud of cigarette smoke floated against the foam tile ceiling and green fluorescent lights. A few people playing cards stopped to look at me. The foyer behind them opened into a room with couches and ashtrays and dingy blue curtains that framed a window hazy from years of weather and cigarette smoke. Metal screens obscured the view outside.

Sam walked to what looked like a drive-through window and spoke to someone inside. A lock clicked and a woman stepped out from the nurses' station.

"How about a tour of the unit?" she asked.

Sam stayed behind while Mom and I followed the woman to the nearest bedroom. Two plain wooden beds covered in blue hospital quilts sat side by side about five feet apart. A middle-aged man went about his business, walking in and out of the bathroom as if he were getting ready to go to work. The woman introduced the two of us. We were going to be roommates, she said. I went to shake his hand and he said we weren't allowed to touch anyone.

Mom and I followed the woman out of the bedroom and down the hallway into a small dining area. Two short lines of tables and chairs occupied most of the space.

"This is where you'll eat," the woman said. "There's a microwave for you to use, and plates and utensils are in the cabinets and drawers next to it."

Mom and I followed her back to the nurses' station. Sam was standing inside. I watched him through the window as he wrote in a large book with a blue plastic cover.

Sam moved around the office with a confident familiarity. He knew which drawers held which items. He spoke to staff in a casual, acquainted voice. His gestures were relaxed and easy. The woman handed me a few papers as I watched him.

He knows this place, I thought. *He's done this before.*

I'd never doubted Sam. I'd always believed he cared about me. He understood why I liked punk rock, and he never bad-mouthed my clothes or friends. But for the first time, as I stood there watching him, I wondered if he had just betrayed me.

"You'll need to read those," the woman said, tapping the papers.

The handout looked like a vocabulary assignment. Terms were printed in one column and definitions in the other. Phrases like "Suicide Precaution (SP)" and "Combative Precaution (CP)" filled the page.

Sam finished his paperwork and then stepped out of the office. The door locked with a click behind him. "Banning, I'll be back to see you again tomorrow." He turned to my mom. "Do you have a few minutes, Valerie?"

"It's going to be okay," Mom said to me.

I gave her a hug, fighting a childish urge to hold on.

"I love you, honey," she said. "I'll be back soon."

Mom followed Sam to the double doors at the front of the unit. The nurse escorting us slid a key into a small metal panel nearby. The lock clicked and Sam pushed the door open for my mother. I watched as they stepped into the elevator-sized space. Mom turned to look at me through one of the narrow wire-reinforced windows in the doors. She waved and silently mouthed the words "I love you."

Then they left.

3

A Sick Game of Twister

Unit B contained one TV, several decks of cards, a double-sided chess and checkerboard, and about twenty chain-smoking adults. I was one of two teenagers. The other, a guy named Mal, left three days after I arrived. Most of the adults treated me like an innocent child. They taught me gin rummy, spades, and the Serenity Prayer. The first time I said I wanted to go home, one of the patients, a middle-aged guy who used his AA sobriety chips to play poker, reminded me I'd been placed on a short-term unit for adults.

"But I'm fifteen," I said.

"I wouldn't worry about it," he told me, his cigarette bobbing in rhythm with his lower lip. "A couple of weeks and you'll be out."

I met my assigned doctor the morning after my admission. Dr. Anderson was a short man with pale skin and the teeth of a rodent. He only smiled when he disagreed with me. Our relationship consisted of brief transactions where he asked me questions while taking notes in the same blue-covered chart Sam had been writing in the day before.

"So it says here you gave your skateboard away," he said.

"Yeah, because my friend broke his, but I bought a new one."

"It also states that you . . ." He watched his finger as he followed it across the page. "Told a friend of yours that everyone would be better off without you around." He looked at me again. "Is that true?"

"I guess," I said. "But I've said that to my mom a million times. Half my friends say it too and they're not in here."

"Have you been depressed lately?"

"No."

"You aren't sad about your parents' divorce?" he asked.

"Well, sure, I guess. But this is all a mistake."

He raised an eyebrow. "A mistake?"

I sat upright in my chair and spoke slowly, as if he hadn't understood me. "I gave my skateboard to a friend, but I bought a new one. So yes, this is all a mistake."

I was fifteen. I didn't know if I was depressed. I knew I was tired of being hurt and I missed my friends and I wanted a family. But Dr. Anderson never asked what I wanted. Instead, he ordered a series of tests for me. The next day I spent hours filling out something called an MMPI and looking at ink blots that looked like bats, moths, and pressed leaves. Twice a day I attended a group meeting where people discussed addiction and eating disorders. On the few occasions I mentioned my parents' divorce, people nodded silently. My problems felt small compared with theirs. The only exception seemed to be the place where I was being held.

"They won't let me go outside," I told Sam later that week. "I can't use the phone or call my friends. We can't even touch anybody, like no hugs or anything."

"Dr. Anderson's still reviewing your case, but I'll be coming to see you once a week."

One week passed. Then two. I kept my things packed and ready in my closet. But no matter how many times I asked Sam or the staff if my mom had made plans to pick me up, they always told me to talk to Dr. Anderson.

I had only gotten to know a few people in my first two weeks on unit B. The twenty or so patients were an ever-changing mixture of adults and the occasional teenager, like Mal. Unit A, one of the neighboring wings, was dedicated to alcoholism. Units C and D were for adolescents. Everyone spoke of unit C differently, though. People whispered stories about kids who had been there for months or years. There were even rumors that some of them had been tied to beds. The few occasions I heard unit C mentioned left me wondering what terrible things really happened there. And with each passing day I grew more afraid of what everyone called "the adolescent long-term unit."

I was only allowed to see my mom once a week, and I always made sure to find a quiet corner of the dayroom where I could beg her to take me home.

"I don't want to be here anymore," I told her. "I hate it here. It's depressing. They won't even let me go outside."

Mom patted my knee. "Sam said they're almost done with your evaluation. It'll only be a few more days."

Before I'd been locked in the hospital, all I cared about was music and skating. Now I couldn't even remember the last time I'd knelt in the dirt or touched a tree. Some nights I'd lie in bed and stare at the screened window and imagine I could see the moon and stars. The outdoors had been a part of my life for as long as I could remember. Now it was a just blurry image outside my screened window.

One evening, during one of Mom's visits, my stomach began to cramp. She said I should go ask for some fruit, so I went to the nurses' station and asked for a banana. The nurse handed me an orange.

"Sorry, that's all we have," she said.

After eating only a few slices, I began to feel worse. Mom and I wrapped up our visit, and when I told the nurse I still didn't feel well, she gave me some milk of magnesia and told me to go to bed.

I woke in the middle of the night in gut-wrenching pain. My roommate had been discharged days before, so I tried calling out for help when a surge of thick, bitter fluid rose in my throat. I crawled to the bathroom before vomiting on the floor and passing out. The next thing I remember was being carried back to my bed. Staff laid me flat and I screamed in agony. I couldn't straighten my body. I had to curl up in a ball, and even that was excruciating.

Several people were standing over my bed when a nurse said she needed to take my blood. She wiped my forearm with alcohol and drew a couple of vials and then hurried away. Another nurse came in to watch me until the doctor returned. She was young and had black hair and she held my hand on her knees while she explained immune responses and white blood cell counts. It was the first time in weeks that someone seemed to truly care about me. I could have listened to her for hours, but the doctor came back and interrupted her. He said my appendix needed to come out immediately. Staff brought a gurney and placed it next to my bed and warned me to brace myself. Then they counted to three and lifted me. I shrieked in pain. They rolled me out of my room and the doors clicked and the nurses rushed me through the hospital, headfirst, the world in reverse. Then a doctor asked me to count backward from ten. I made it to seven.

My eyes were closed when I grew conscious. The room was bright and I could hear birds singing. I cracked my eyes to see a window without a security screen. The world outside was clear and colorful. A cool breeze drifted through the hair on my arms.

"I had the window open when I held you for the first time in the hospital," Mom said. "I could smell the ocean." She stood up from a chair in the corner and smiled at me. "How are you feeling, honey?"

I struggled to get a better look out the window. "Can I go outside?"

Mom grinned and nodded. "You'll have to take it easy for a day or two, though." She said my appendix had almost ruptured. The incision was enormous, about five inches long, and stapled shut. Other than being forced to cough every hour, I loved being in a real hospital. The nurses let me listen to music and watch TV. I could open my window whenever I wanted, even in the middle of the night. Sometimes I'd hang my head outside and stare at the stars. One morning I hobbled downstairs so I could stand in the sunlight and feel the crisp winter air. People smiled as they walked past, staring at me dressed in my hospital gown while I gazed at the sky. The world seemed different now, more beautiful. I didn't want to lose it again.

Dad came to see me the day after my surgery. He walked into my room wearing his uniform and said he was in town on a flight. I felt like I was eight years old again, small and fragile and awestruck.

"How are you feeling?" he asked, setting down his flight case.

"I'm okay."

"Sounds like your appendix almost ruptured."

"I guess. That's what the doctors said."

"You know, Jeff Farrell had his appendix out just a few days before his Olympic swim trials," he said. "A few weeks later he got a gold medal."

I stared at him for a moment, dumbfounded.

"Oh," I said.

Dad fidgeted with his flight cap. He began picking at some invisible piece of lint.

"When am I going home?" I asked. "I don't want to go back to unit B. I hate it there."

"Sam said they're still finishing up the evaluation."

"He said that three weeks ago, when he told me I'd be here for two weeks."

Dad turned and walked to the window. I could see his reflection in the glass.

"Adrienne's studying to become a doctor," he said, changing the subject. "She came home to visit the other day. And you should see the house. I'm working on a guest room above the barn."

My dad seemed unable to believe that he had made a mistake, that all of this was happening because he had sent me away. He had done the same thing when he left me at the airport. He just handed me some money and told me to call my mom and then walked away. I'd never felt real anger toward my dad, but that day I wanted to scream at him, the same way punk rock had screamed at me about being let down and betrayed by people. Instead, I leaned back in the hospital bed and let him keep talking about himself and Linda and the house, until he finally ran out of things to say. Then there was a long pause and he walked back to his flight case and put on his cap.

"I guess I should get going," he said.

"Already?"

"I'm heading back home early in the morning. I traded a trip just so I could see you."

I wondered if I would ever understand my father. My entire perspective on him consisted of childhood memories I had pieced together to try to understand why he didn't want me anymore. From the moment I first knew he was a pilot, I wanted to be like him. I'd memorized every plane in the black-and-white photographs that used to hang in our house. When I was in kindergarten, I brought him as my show-and-tell assignment so he could talk to my class about being a pilot. My dad was the center of my universe when I was a kid. Now that he was married to Linda, he seemed like a stranger.

He picked up his flight case and then shook my hand. I watched him as if I were recording the moment on a tape in my mind, reminding myself that the love I felt was for someone else, the man who used to introduce me to his friends and walk me down the aisle to my seat, with his hat perched on my head like I was the king of the world.

But that man was gone now. As far as I was concerned, my dad was dead.

Dr. Anderson asked to see me the morning after I returned from the hospital. He led me to a small examination room and closed the door.

The room's dim fluorescent lighting made him look stranger than usual. He opened my chart and skimmed its pages. He said he had been reviewing the results of my tests.

"Apparently you've had a difficult time making friends since your parents' divorce," he said.

I'm in here because I gave my skateboard to a friend, you fucking asshole. What don't you understand?

He scanned a few more lines, then stopped and tapped one of them as if he had suddenly found something interesting. "These results are symptomatic of someone who suffers from major depression," he said. I mumbled something about not being depressed and he stopped reading and looked at me. His teeth appeared small and green in the dim lighting. He smiled and tapped the page again.

"Yes, but you're also suffering from denial," he said.

I'd had some doubts about Sam, but he never treated me like I was broken. He was always kind to me. And now that I'd been cut off from my friends and the outside world, he was the only friend I had left.

Dr. Anderson closed my chart and watched me for a moment before he spoke again.

"Since unit B's unable to offer you a stable environment or peers your age, I believe it would be in your best interest to have you transferred to unit C, the adolescent long-term unit."

The room seemed to spin for a moment. Then there was nothing, just a blinding panic that made everything seem dim and far away. I don't recall Dr. Anderson leaving the room. I only remember the bright light from the hallway as he opened the door, and the cool air drifting over my sweaty face as I wandered back to my room and sat on the foot of my bed.

———

My remaining days on unit B were numb and distant. I watched myself get out of bed, sit in group meetings, and then go back to my room and lie in the darkness, only to wake up and repeat the same day over again until the night of my transfer. I remember standing near the nurses' station, holding two shopping bags full of my belongings. The dinner cart was still in the hallway and the dayroom smelled like fish sticks and cigarettes. A small group of patients waved to me from nearby. Their smiles looked fragile and worried.

"Remember, no hugs," one of the staff said.

The doors clicked and unlocked. Two staff members escorted me off the unit and across the rotunda to face a nearly identical locked entrance. My shoes had been taken from me so I couldn't run, and the carpet outside the doors felt cold beneath my feet.

One of the staff pressed a button on the wall. I looked through the wire-reinforced windows to see an empty hallway. The unit looked abandoned.

A man with a small black mustache and glasses stepped out of a room inside the unit. He unlocked the doors and pushed one open.

"I'm Luther, one of the staff here on unit C," the man said.

He took a wire-tethered key from his belt and inserted it into a metal panel on the wall. The inner doors unlocked and he pushed one of them open before stepping in front of me and starting down the hallway. The doors clicked and locked behind us.

Unit C was meticulously clean and smelled of sweet cinnamon disinfectant. There were no tables full of people or games of gin rummy. No conversations or laughter. An unsettling stillness permeated the place, as if something terrible lived in one of the rooms that no one wanted to awaken.

I followed Luther down the hallway toward the nurses' station. His black thick-soled shoes never made a sound. After a few steps we passed the entrance to the dayroom, where more than a dozen teenagers were gathered on sofas arranged in a loose circle. A woman in her forties sat among the group. She was pretty, with long black hair and olive skin. She wore an ankle-length skirt suit and heels. She watched me for a moment, wearing a subtle, indecipherable smile on her face before turning back to the group. A young girl was crying. She lowered her head to hide her face behind a curtain of long brown hair. A few kids looked at me. The others appeared so absorbed in whatever had happened that they didn't seem to realize I was there.

Then I noticed a wheeled bed in the corner of the dayroom. A young girl lay on it, watching me. Tangled, dirty black hair surrounded her face like a cloud of flies. Thick leather cuffs bound her wrists and ankles, and long straps held her legs spread-eagle. She craned her neck to watch me, her unblinking black eyes following me as if she were pleading for help.

They really do tie people to beds.

I staggered to the nurses' station. A woman inside took my belongings and said she'd return them later. Luther told me to follow him into a nearby bedroom.

"I'll need some of my things for bed," I said.

"You'll get them back once we determine what needs to be locked in your closet and what you can keep. You and your roommate are both on SPs," he said, referring to suicide precautions. "Anything you or your roommate can use to hurt yourselves will be locked in the closet or given to your parents to take home. Pens, pencils, shoelaces, things like that."

Voices in the dayroom broke into murmured conversations.

"Sounds like the unit meeting's ending now. Be right back." Luther stepped into the hallway and spoke to someone. "No talking," he said.

There was a mechanical clicking sound followed by a loud voice and laughter. A kid tied to a wheelchair rolled into the room. He looked younger than me, with a short black afro and a huge grin.

"Hey, I'm Michael," he said.

He had been tied to his wheelchair using the same straps as the girl I'd seen minutes before, but they had been loosened so he could roll himself around without assistance. He was bright and animated and happily wheeled himself around the room while he got ready for bed. Sometimes Luther would lengthen one of his belt-like arm or leg restraints so he could brush his teeth or stand up to use the sink, but the leather cuffs binding each of his wrists and ankles never came off.

Once Michael finished getting ready for the night, Luther stepped into the hallway to ask for assistance. Then he and another staff member guided Michael through something like a sick game of Twister, slowly transferring each of Michael's cuffed limbs from his wheelchair to his bed while making sure to unlock only one strap at a time. Five minutes later the process was complete, and Michael, still smiling, had been secured for the evening.

The moment Luther and his partner left the room, Michael turned to look at me.

"Mind if I fart?" he said.

I stared at him. He chuckled and farted. We both burst into laughter. Michael appeared to be a typical teenager, although he didn't seem to care that he had been tied to a bed. I had so many questions for him. *What did you do? Why are you here? Why are you tied to a bed?* Instead, I asked the first question that wasn't personal.

"Who's that girl that was . . ."

"That's Sonia," he said, staring at the ceiling.

"How long has she been in restraints?"

Michael shrugged. "A long time, I guess. Before I got here."

I was about to ask how long he had been on the unit when there was a knock on our open door. A stern, round-faced woman walked into our room. "Time for your meds, Michael," she said. She handed him a tiny paper cup. The pills inside rattled as he threw back his head and tossed them into his mouth. Then, reaching up with his leather-cuffed arm tethered to a barely lengthened strap, he took a small cup of water from her and grimaced before swallowing the medication.

He opened his mouth and groaned a long, single note. "Ahh . . ."

She peered inside and asked him to lift his tongue and then left the room.

"Why'd she look in your mouth?" I said.

"To make sure I'm not hiding any pills."

"Why would you do that?"

"Some people save 'em up for later," he said. "That way they can take 'em all at once and try to kill themselves."

I laughed. I thought he was joking. It turned out he wasn't.

4

The Chair

Unit C severed my last few connections to reality. There were no televisions or radios or games of gin rummy. Every night I fell asleep to the sound of kids tapping in code on the walls because talking was forbidden after lights-out. Quiet laughter from bedrooms was chased down by staff looking for those responsible. During one of our unit meetings, a blond girl from Louisiana burst into tears. "I don't want to go home," she said. "I don't know how to live out there anymore." Everyone nodded in sympathy while I sat there awestruck, wondering why anyone would want to stay. She had been in the hospital for three years. A week later a guy with dark brown eyes snuck into a girl's bedroom, and we all woke the next morning to find him tied to a bed. Another girl was told to stop chewing gum. When she refused, a group of staff members strapped her to a wheelchair. Every day I crawled out of bed smaller and more terrified than the day before.

Until my parents signed me in to the hospital, my life had almost no structure. My mom was rarely home, and I spent most days doing whatever I wanted, usually skating or hanging out with my friends. Now my entire life had been reduced to a schedule on a whiteboard that hung near the entrance to the dayroom. We were given half an hour to wake up and get dressed and ready. Half an hour to eat breakfast in a small room where we all sat at tables and shoveled cold cereal into our mouths under the supervision of staff. We spent the rest of the morning in school. Then we got an hour for lunch before going back to class. We had a unit meeting after school, followed by half an hour of group therapy supervised by one of the doctors. Then an hour or two for one of the various activities that staff called AT, OT, and RT, which stood for art, occupational, and recreational therapy. Art therapy meant finger painting or arranging some flowers in a crumbly block of green foam. Occupational therapy required filling out worksheets, crosswords, or other activities. Recreational therapy consisted of push-ups, sit-ups, and jumping jacks in the hallway, which seemed pointless because half a dozen kids on the unit were strapped to wheelchairs or beds, while the rest of us had been locked inside for so long that two minutes of exercise left us all gasping for breath.

Unit meetings were exhausting. The hour-long gatherings required us to sit in the dayroom and talk under the supervision of staff or the occasional doctor. Before my transfer, the groups had been a twice-a-day occurrence. But on unit C we spent as many as four or five hours a day in unit meetings or therapy. Anyone who didn't speak was interrogated for avoiding their issues or being in denial. Those who did speak often broke down in tears. Staff and doctors challenged people to talk about things they had shared with them in private. I had been on the unit for less than a month when staff confronted a fourteen-year-old girl who had confided in them that she had a crush on me. "I think you need to share your feelings with him," one of them said. The girl began to cry and pulled her hair over her face. Everyone fell silent. Someone passed her a box of tissue. I wanted to crawl into a hole and disappear. Staff kept urging her to speak until she finally broke down and admitted her feelings to me. She didn't speak in another unit meeting for days.

My rodent-like physician from the previous unit didn't attend unit C. Instead, the doctor assigned to me was the black-haired woman I'd seen among the kids on my first night. During her daily rounds, Dr. Fisher often pulled me out of unit meetings or found me sitting on a disciplinary "thirty-minute chair" in the hallway because I'd forgotten to close my door. Almost everything about her was pleasant and attractive, from her soft southern accent to her mysterious smile. But after two weeks on the unit, I didn't trust her—or anyone else.

"Sitting chair" was agonizing. Some days I'd spend more than four hours sitting in the hallway outside my door. I'd always been active and restless, and keeping my feet flat on the floor with my hands in my lap for thirty minutes seemed impossible. After three weeks I'd collected dozens of demerits called "test marks," for everything from slouching in my chair to talking after lights-out, so Dr. Fisher ordered staff to put me on "indefinite chair," leaving me to sit in silence when other kids were given free time to play board games in the dayroom.

The only time I was allowed off my chair, other than unit meetings, group therapy, and bedtime, was during school. Twice a week my district sent a teacher to help me with my freshman classes. She was an older woman, quiet and kind, and we'd sit together in my room and go through my lessons for a few precious hours. I spent the other three days of the week doing homework with the rest of the kids in a secure classroom that bordered our unit.

I'd been on unit C for a month when Dr. Fisher peered around the corner of the dayroom during a unit meeting and gestured for me to follow her. She always held our private sessions in the room I shared with Michael. I sat on my bed as she closed the door and turned off the lights. She dragged over the chair from my desk and sat before crossing her legs and then smoothing the wrinkles out of her long pink skirt.

"Staff tell me you're having a difficult time remembering to close your door," she said.

"I don't get why I'm supposed to close it. There's nothing to steal in here."

"It's for everyone's safety. You were given plenty of thirty-minute chairs to consider why, and you've collected quite a few test marks for acting out. Staff noted in your chart you've received test marks for talking, making eye contact, and laughing with others. Then you were finally put on indefinite chair." Dr. Fisher lowered her voice. "Do you think closing your door is the real issue? Or do you think something else is causing you to act out?"

My heart stopped. The doctors and staff often mentioned "not being able to control yourself" or "acting out" whenever they tied someone to a bed or wheelchair. They said restraints were "intended to help" us, but it always felt more like a threat.

Just cooperate, I thought. *Try to figure out what she wants to hear.*

"I guess I should use my chair time to focus on how I'm feeling or what I'm avoiding," I said. "Maybe it's an opportunity instead of a punishment."

A vague smile curled the edges of Dr. Fisher's lips. I couldn't exactly interpret the expression, but from what I could tell it meant I'd done something right.

Sam still came to see me once or twice a week. He always arrived wearing a grin and one of his shiny polyester suits, complete with cowboy boots and bolo. I wanted to hate him for telling my parents to sign me in to the hospital, but he was my only connection to the world outside now. And after two months of isolation, I was lonely. Nearly all of the kids, including me, had been diagnosed with depression, but the staff and doctors never let us go outside or hug anyone. But Sam wasn't like the other doctors. He even moved differently. He'd slouch in his chair during our sessions and prop his feet on my bed. He looked like a cartoon character compared with the doctors and staff. I wasn't sure if I could trust him completely, but I knew he wouldn't put me in restraints if I complained about being in a psych ward. Our weekly sessions were the only time I felt safe. He seemed more like a friend than a therapist now.

I spent most of our weekly sessions talking about how much I missed the outdoors, so he began committing the last fifteen minutes of our time together to a guided meditation of my memory of the world outside. I'd sit on my bed and close my eyes and share a favorite memory of sailing or hiking with my dad, like the time we knelt in the dirt together to look at a millipede, or when we anchored in a harbor near Catalina to spend the night before sailing home in the morning.

One day, after arriving for one of our sessions, Sam closed the door to my room and turned my chair backward and sat facing me with his arms propped on the backrest.

"How're you doing?" he asked.

"Everyone says they're sad because I replaced some girl named Jennifer," I said. She'd left unit C shortly before my transfer. "I feel like shit. I'm just starting to make some friends, but people keep bringing her up. That's all we do in here, talk about the same shit over and over. And if people don't talk, then staff make them."

Sam nodded.

"And how is being locked in here all day and sitting in a chair good for me?" I said. "I never get to go outside. No one in here's happy. Every time we laugh, staff tell us we're acting out. People even cry about being forced to leave because their insurance is running out. It's crazy. One girl's been in here for three years. I can't do that, Sam. I'll go fucking nuts. I'd be eighteen when I left."

I fell quiet and stared out the screened window. Sam leaned to the side and shifted in his chair, the way people do when they're about to change the subject.

"Dr. Fisher tells me they've put you on indefinite chair," he said. "She mentioned you keep leaving your door open."

"I'm in a fucking psych ward, Sam. There's nothing to steal in here. I don't get the whole 'It's for patient safety' thing. Wouldn't it be safer to keep our doors *open* so you could see if someone's hiding in their room or something?"

He shrugged. "It's not my rule. Agree or disagree, it's one you're supposed to follow."

I looked back out the window. The woven metal screen outside left the image blurry and confused. I stared at the screen for a long time before I spoke again.

"I miss going out there," I said. "I miss the smell of the rain and the way trees sound in the wind. I miss skating with my friends after school. I miss seeing the sky and the stars and sleeping with my window open so I can listen to the crickets at night."

Sam watched me and smiled. He shifted in his chair again.

"Do you like reading?" he asked.

"I guess. I liked *Great Expectations*, and I read a couple of Ray Bradbury's short stories when I was in junior high."

"What about *Jonathan Livingston Seagull*?"

The name evoked a memory of seeing it on a shelf. "No, but I think my mom has it."

"I'll have her bring it for you," Sam said. "I think you'd like it."

"When am I going to find time to read? All I do is sit chair."

"Doesn't a teacher come from your district to help you with your schoolwork?" he asked.

"Yeah, but she's only here a couple of times a week."

"I bet she'd be happy to help you find time to read," Sam said. "I'll leave a note for her."

I devoured the book in days, so Sam asked Dr. Fisher to approve a few others by Ernest Hemingway. Mom began bringing me a new book every week. I cherished all of them, with their stories and people and places so different from the prison that had become my home.

———

Days later I was sitting in my normal spot outside my door when someone in the hallway began to laugh. Luther stepped out of the nurses' station. His small brown eyes scanned the three or four of us sitting in the
hallway.

"That's a test mark, Banning," he said.

"For what?"

"You're distracting Kevin."

Kevin had been in the hospital for nearly two years. He had spent
more than a month in restraints. He always sat in the hallway about ten
feet to my right, shackled to his wheelchair next to the entrance to his
room. He was thin and delicate, almost elfin, and his hair seemed to
naturally shape itself into a messy Elvis-style pompadour. He didn't often speak in group, but I remember him saying he'd been picked on for
being gay and that he had an eating disorder.

"Test marks for everyone! King Luther commands it!" Kevin said in
the high-pitched voice of Fred, his fictitious imaginary friend. A moment
later, in his normal voice, he responded to himself. "But Fred, we don't
want test marks. Test marks are bad."

"That's one for you too," Luther said to him.

Kevin frowned and slumped in his wheelchair like Pinocchio. As Luther turned to leave, Kevin sat up and raised his loosely tethered hand.

"Wait. I have a question," he said.

Luther turned to look at him. "Yes?"

"Who gets the test mark? Me or Fred?"

Kevin and I burst into laughter. Luther ignored us and then stepped into the nurses' station and announced bedtime. Kevin wheeled himself into his room while the rest of us began getting ready for bed. I was brushing my teeth when Luther walked into our room to adjust Michael's bed restraints.

"Banning, you've been acting out since the day you arrived," Luther said. "Why are you so defiant? Staff thinks it's a call for help."

I mumbled through my toothpaste. "How is laughing or slouching in my chair a call for help?"

"Because we've asked you to stop, and you refuse."

Michael glared at me from his bed and shook his head.

Don't respond. That's what Luther wants.

Luther turned to leave and then stopped to finish a thought. "Banning, if we ask you to sit up straight, and you refuse, then I'd say you can't control yourself." He stepped out of sight before reappearing a moment later with my blue-covered chart. My name was written on the spine, last name first. We all wondered about our charts. They held a sort of mystical awe, as if each handwritten word detailed the darkest secrets of our mental illness.

Luther pulled up a chair and sat outside our doorway and watched me get ready for bed while he scribbled notes on one of the pages. He stayed there after lights-out, his silhouette still writing, while Michael lay five feet away from me, tied to his bed as he stared at the ceiling.

It was sometime the next week when I returned to my chair after one of my sessions with Dr. Fisher. Our meetings seemed pointless. No matter what I shared with her or how honestly I tried to express my feelings, nothing ever seemed to change. I'd been confined to my chair for weeks because I'd forgotten to close the door to my room. After I remembered to close my door, she said I had to keep sitting chair because I'd gotten test marks for slouching or laughing. Then, when I finally started cooperating, she said I was being too compliant and wasn't taking therapy seriously. None of it made any sense. Dr. Fisher said I was depressed, but she made me sit in a chair in the hallway. She said I had a hard time making friends, but she said I couldn't hug anyone or have any private conversations. Staff told us to share our feelings, but they tied kids to beds for raising their voices or getting upset. How was I supposed to take therapy seriously when it looked and felt like abuse?

Instead, I began treating the hospital like a puzzle. I analyzed everything. The way Dr. Fisher would slowly nod when I used certain phrases. The way Luther grinned at someone when they agreed with him. How the kids who left the soonest talked a little bit but never too much. Everything became a puzzle I needed to solve. And everyone became a part of it, even the friends I was still getting to know.

There were a few of those friends, the ones who had been in the hospital the longest, who seemed to have given up trying to make sense of anything. And for some of them, making people laugh was the only way they could deal with our isolation.

"Psst," Kevin whispered one afternoon, sitting in his wheelchair next to the entrance to his room. "Check it out. I'm Luther, Dr. Fisher's little puppet."

Kevin began convulsing in his wheelchair like a marionette. The buckles of his restraints rattled on the wheels. Luther stepped out of the nurses' station and leaned against the wall.

"You know what I'm going to say," he told me.

I almost jumped out of my chair. "What did I do now?"

"You're laughing."

"But he's the one doing it."

"That's another for arguing with me," Luther said. "And a third for not having your feet on the floor."

Kevin began convulsing again. "Hur, hur, hur. That's a test mark. I'm Luther. That's a test mark."

Sonia, tied to her bed and stationed in the hallway for observation, started laughing.

"And that's one for you," Luther said to her.

She rolled her eyes. "Fuck you, Luther. Go back to drawing pictures of you fucking your mom."

Luther ignored her and disappeared into the nurses' station. He hadn't been gone more than ten seconds when Sonia began to sing.

"They say it's your birthday!"

I turned to see her bobbing her head in rhythm to the Beatles' song, her matted black hair swaying around like a tangled bundle of wire. A dozen leather restraints peered out from the edges of the white sheet that covered her body. Bandages protected her wrists and ankles where the restraints had rubbed them raw.

Luther called her name through the nurses' station window. She ignored him.

"They say it's your birthday!"

"Sonia."

"We're gonna have a good time!"

Then a different voice, like a woman paging someone in an airport, spoke over the public address system. "Dr. Rush to unit C. Dr. Rush to unit C."

"Oh, fuck you, Luther!" Sonia yelled. "Calling in your peons. You're a fucking pussy."

I looked at Kevin. He sat still and stared at his knees, like a child pretending to be invisible. Sonia began tugging at her restraints. Kevin closed his eyes.

"You should just lie down, Sonia," Luther said.

"Fuck you, Luther! You're a fucking piece of shit."

She craned her neck and looked at the windowed doors of the unit, where a group of men had already assembled outside the entrance. Down the hall, one of the kids peered around the corner of their doorway. She disappeared into their room and whispered to her roommate, "Sonia's getting rushed."

Luther strolled out of the nurses' station and walked to the foot of Sonia's bed. "Let's get you in your room."

"Get the fuck away from me!" she screamed, lunging for him as her arms strained against her restraints.

The security doors flew open. The men outside sprinted past me and Kevin, their keys jangling in their pockets as they ran. Luther guided Sonia's bed through her doorway while the orderlies held down her arms and legs.

"Get the fuck off of me!" she yelled. "Someone help me!"

The group disappeared into Sonia's room. She began shrieking as the door closed behind them. The woman's voice spoke over the public address system again. More urgent this time. "Dr. Rush to unit C. Stat." Kevin curled up in his wheelchair and covered his ears. The security doors clicked and opened as more orderlies ran into the unit. I closed my eyes as they sprinted down the hallway and into Sonia's bedroom. Through the wall, her disembodied screams sounded like a girl being attacked in a basement.

I sat there for two hours, listening to her cry for help while I stared at the floor or closed my eyes. Sometimes she'd fall quiet and I could hear someone talking to her. Then she'd start yelling at them and they'd tell her to calm down and she'd start fighting again until they called for help and the orderlies brought more restraints.

For months I'd watched them antagonize Sonia. Luther or someone else would prod her with questions or deny her something simple. A crayon or a piece of paper. Then she'd lose her temper and they'd call for Dr. Rush and the orderlies would pour into her room and pin her down and add more restraints. I imagined running into her room and saving her. Sometimes I'd daydream about attacking the nurses and staff, punching and kicking them and then stealing their keys and freeing all of us, wheeling everyone in restraints out through the lobby and into the sunlight so all the normal people outside would see us and say, "Where have you been? Who's done this to you?" And we'd all point at the doctors and staff and then the police would come and take them away.

But I knew I couldn't do anything. I was helpless now, and imagining saving Sonia gave birth to a rage so enormous that it began to suffocate me. She would scream and I'd feel it start clawing its way out of my chest like some alien parasite driven by hatred and revenge. There were times when I thought I'd snap and attack Luther and wind up in restraints like Michael and Kevin and Sonia. I was a captive animal now, a hostage to my helplessness and rage. Even worse, I was a coward. I was so afraid to stand up to Luther and the staff that I buried that rage under the rest of the burning wreckage inside me. And instead of bolting into Sonia's room and trying to free her, I sat in my chair and listened to my heart pounding in my ears until she was too exhausted to scream anymore.

Two hours later, after the staff in the hallway said Sonia had finally fallen asleep, the only thing I could hear was the sound of people crying in their rooms.

By the end of March, Dr. Fisher had ordered my "indefinite chair" to be changed to "permanent chair in room," leaving me to sit in my bedroom, facing the wall, for nearly six hours a day. She announced the change during one of the Saturday morning unit meetings the staff and doctors used to award and revoke privileges. The new restriction also required me to eat alone in my bedroom and effectively removed all my remaining privileges.

"Permanent chair in room" reduced my existence to a still life of a kid imprisoned in a twisted diorama. Every day I sat in a chair facing a pastel wall in a small, dimly lit box, like a wax exhibit in a museum. There was a wooden desk in front of me, two beds behind, and a heavily screened window to my right. There were no paintings, artwork, or decorations. There were no fake plants or trees. No fresh air or weather. No stars or moon. I never felt the sun on my skin or heard crickets at night. Every day featured the same sights and smells. The temperature never changed. Only rarely could I hear anything from outside the walls of the unit. My senses had grown so hungry that when staff came in for a shift change, I could smell rain or sweat on their clothing, even from a distance.

I began studying everyone more closely, especially the kids about to be discharged from the unit. What did they talk about in meetings? Did they smile? Did they cry? Were they confident or vulnerable? For weeks

I took mental notes of the staff, the doctors, and even my friends, watching every tear and smile and uncomfortable laugh to figure out the key to going home. I'd tried everything else. I'd closed my door and talked about my parents and feelings like the other kids, but nothing ever changed. The only way to leave, it seemed, had something to do with insurance. When someone announced they were leaving, they usually said the same thing, "My insurance is pulling me, but I don't want to leave." Some of them, like the pretty girl from Louisiana, had been in the hospital for years.

It wasn't the first time I'd wondered about the people who wanted to stay in the hospital. No one seemed happy. Everyone hated it here, even the girl from Louisiana. But instead of begging to go home, they usually begged to stay.

What's wrong with these people? We're not allowed to go outside, be alone, or even have a hug. Why would anyone want to stay here?

One of the least unpleasant staff members was a man named Charles. He was a tall man with wiry black hair and a bushy mustache. He was also the first to notice I always tipped my chair backward and rocked in place. He made a habit of pointing it out to me with irritating regularity. So when he peered around the corner of my doorway one day and pointed at the floor, I grinned and lowered my chair to the ground.

"You gotta stop rocking your chair," he said. "If you keep it up, you're gonna wear a hole in the carpet."

Charles hadn't been gone ten seconds by the time I'd tipped my chair backward and started rocking again. I didn't even notice I'd done it until I heard a sigh of disappointment from the doorway. I turned to see Luther watching me.

"Charles just asked you to stop rocking your chair," he said. "And I'm giving you a second test mark for not sitting up straight."

They'll put me in restraints if I keep getting test marks.

Luther walked away and I returned my gaze to the familiar patch of wall in front of me. For weeks I'd daydreamed while I stared at its textured surface, imagining its strange landscape as continents of a distant planet or the surface of the moon. But that day, as my mind returned to wandering those imaginary lands, with its hills and valleys and wild places far away, I suddenly realized I'd started rocking my chair again.

I'm not a fucking animal. I know I can control myself.

I shoved myself upright and fixed my eyes on the wall and then pushed my spine into the chair until its barely upholstered back dug under my shoulder blades.

For the next two hours I gazed at the wall while my mind roamed from one memory to the next. Then someone would cough or a door would click and my mind would scurry back to the present. I began reciting a single word in a low whisper, barely loud enough to hear. "Focus." But my mind refused to obey. I'd recall sailing with my dad or skateboarding down an alley on a cold winter morning, and then out of the sky or sea or wherever my memory had taken me, the word would repeat itself, like a voice from an angry god. "Focus."

What's wrong with me? I thought. *This is my mind. These are my thoughts.*

I fixed my eyes on the wall again and repeated my mantra, but my body grew sore and restless in its stillness. I'd start bouncing my leg or rocking my chair, only to notice minutes later that I was staring out the window. The image through the screen in our bedroom had been my only view of the world for months. And after spending hundreds of hours staring at the wall, I often found the temptation to look outside too powerful to resist. But the tightly woven metal screen was so dense that looking outside meant staring at more screen than scenery, giving the image behind it the appearance of a painting in pointillism. Soon I discovered that if I tipped my chair backward and swayed, as if I were sitting in a rocking chair, the screen would disappear and leave the scene outside clear and sharp.

"Banning, I asked you earlier to keep your chair on the floor."

I turned to see Luther staring at me from the doorway again. He leaned against the wall like a guy taking a cigarette break with a coworker. I held his gaze for a moment and then looked at the wall before lowering the legs of my chair to the carpet.

"Sometimes I wonder why you're so defiant," he said. "The doctors and staff know you can do better. We're only trying to help you."

Oh, fuck you, Luther.

"Maybe it's a call for help," I said, lying. "Trusting people is hard for me."

"It's hard for a lot of folks. But help requires trust. Don't you trust us?"

"I think so. Sometimes I do," I lied again. "It's just scary. I think some part of me resents therapy, which is probably why I'm on chair, so I can figure that stuff out."

Luther's eyes widened. "Really? I don't get the impression you're thinking about your issues. All you do is rock back and forth in your chair and stare out the window instead of using your chair time to be productive. Seems to me like you can't control yourself."

He fixed his gaze on me and I looked away. I knew better than to irritate him. Out of the corner of my eye, I watched him lean away from the door, and he paused to look at me a last time before walking back to the nurses' station, his keys jangling quietly as he strolled down the hallway.

The sunlight and shadow in the courtyard outside my window changed with the coming of summer, and with it came the muffled footsteps of work boots overhead. Staff explained the hospital was being expanded and we'd soon be relocated to a new unit upstairs. Every week the sounds changed, from the screeching of drills and saws to the rhythmic thumping of hammers on drywall. Listening to the construction became my favorite pastime while I sat chair. I'd close my eyes and focus on what I could hear of the world above. The distant voices of men and the sound of their radio. Mumbled conversations and laughter. Their tired, heavy strides as they left for the day. I imagined I'd made new friends.

One evening, long after the workers had gone, Michael's therapist arrived for their session. They always used our room, so I dragged my chair into the hallway and settled outside our door.

Bonnie, one of the staff, peered out of the nurses' station. "I told you yesterday, stop scratching your chest, Banning."

I hadn't even noticed I'd done it. I slouched and hung my hands by my sides. The itching returned a moment later and I snuck my hand into my shirt.

"Stop it," Bonnie said. "Come here. Let me take a look."

I stood and stretched my legs before walking to the window of the nurses' station. After months of sitting chair, my body felt fragile and sore.

"What's going on with your chest? Lift your shirt for me."

"Banning's flashing Bonnie!" Sonia shouted from her bed in the hallway. "Call Dr. Rush!"

"Hush it, Sonia," Bonnie said before turning back to me. "You need to stoop down. I'm staring at your belly button."

I bent over and looked down at the top of her head. Her brown hair had turned gray and she'd dyed it a bizarre red color. Her roots were an inch long.

"Yeah, you've got a mole that's irritated," she said. "I'll leave a note in your chart."

Dr. Fisher and I met the following afternoon. She mentioned Bonnie's message about my mole and asked me to take off my shirt. She stepped toward me, backlit against the window, and I held my breath as she leaned forward. My eyes drew a line down her neck. I could see the freckles above the top of her lace-trimmed camisole and the way her breasts gently moved as she breathed. I could smell her hair and the perfume on her blouse. Long, delicate coils of black hair trailed over her shoulders, glistening in sunlight through the window behind her. I hadn't been close to anyone in months.

"It's probably best to have a dermatologist take a look at it," she said. "I'll make a note in your chart and schedule an appointment."

The weeks leading up to that day left me nervous and excited. There had been a long-standing rumor on the unit that going to see any of the specialist physicians meant traveling to the professional building across the street. I spent the morning of my appointment rocking my chair, hoping to catch a glimpse of the weather outside.

Charles peered around the corner of our doorway. "Chair down, please."

"Do I get to walk today?"

"If you're asking if you'll be in wheelchair restraints, you won't," he said. "I'll be escorting you along with someone else."

I sighed and my stomach unknotted itself. For weeks I'd been afraid the appointment would require my being tied to a wheelchair and rolled across the street.

"But we'll need to take your shoes," Charles added. "Just wear your socks."

It was almost noon when he returned. Standing next to him was one of the newer staff members, a younger guy who rarely spoke. I hadn't been outside in over four months, not since my appendectomy, when I used to hobble down to the lobby in my hospital gown and stand in the sunlight and stare at the sky.

I peeled off my shoes and Charles locked them in my closet. Then he escorted me through the inner security doors and waited for the other staff member to step inside. My heart began to race.

"We're just going across the street," Charles said. "No detours." He looked at me and grinned. "Okay?"

The security doors clicked and opened and we stepped into the rotunda. Charles waited for the doors to lock behind us. The world suddenly felt enormous. The air was cool and drifted over my arms and face. Carts rattled down hallways. People hurried from one place to another. Two women stood talking in a doorway nearby and one of them said something and they broke into laughter. I'd forgotten happiness like that, the kind that jumped out of people when they weren't afraid of everything.

Charles led us down a hallway and into a long corridor. The doors at the far end had been propped open and daylight illuminated the walls and tile floor. A light wind drifted over the hair on my arms. The summer air smelled of grass and trees. We neared the end of the hallway as something inside me began to stir to life, awakened by the sunlight and warmth of the world. I stopped in the doorway and shaded my eyes. The sun seemed impossibly bright. The staff member following me put his hand on my shoulder, then carefully guided me forward as I stepped onto the warm concrete.

"Wait a sec," I said. "I can't see."

I caught a glimpse of Charles turning to face me before my eyes forced themselves closed.

Motionless, I stood in a sea of sun-warmed air and sound. Voices no longer echoed. In the absence of walls, words were free to leave. Sparrows flitted in a hedge, bickering and chirping as they chased one another. The soft hum of traffic on the highway murmured in the distance. A flag nearby snapped in the breeze and the rope used to raise it rapped a rhythm on the hollow metal flagpole. The sound reminded me of sailing when I was a child, the way the ropes struck the mast and made it ring like a bell. I pictured sitting on the prow of our tiny boat, the ocean sprawled out in front of me, blue and endless. But this wasn't that world anymore. This was a thousand times more beautiful than the world I remembered.

I cracked my eyes and blinked against the sunlight. Charles was still standing in front of me. Behind him, on the far side of the street, stood a pale brick building bordered by a row of short bushes. I shaded my eyes and looked overhead. Thin wisps of gossamer clouds floated in the sky, like feathers on the surface of a pool.

Charles glanced at the other staff member and grinned. "Let's hold up a sec," he said.

I closed my eyes and lifted my face toward the sky. The sun shone red through my eyelids. I thought of the ocean again, hundreds of miles away, and the mountains near my dad's house in Sonoma, with its valley and vineyards and the mist that hovered over the tall grass in the morning. I drew a long, slow breath from the air, the same air as those faraway places, then held it as I imagined shaping all those things into a beautiful keepsake, like a piece of amber containing the wind, the sky, the sunlight, and its warmth. Then, opening a small door that concealed my heart, I placed that keepsake alongside all my other memories. The moment was mine now and the doctors and staff could never take it away.

5

I Just Want to Go Home

The hospital's expansion was completed in June. One by one we were escorted up the secure fire escape to find a nearly identical prison waiting for us upstairs. Sonia and the few others in restraints were brought up in the elevator and rolled into the dayroom like shackled circus animals. The new unit was spotless. Even the staff seemed impressed. They wandered around with the rest of us, fidgeting with the new door handles and admiring the bright gray industrial carpet and peach-colored walls. After months of living in a run-down psychiatric unit, the smallest improvement in our lives seemed like cause for celebration. Even things as trivial as new light switches and bathrooms felt like novelties.

Days after our relocation, Dr. Fisher summoned me for one of our sessions. I followed her to the new bedroom I shared with Michael and she turned off the lights and sat with my chart in her lap.

"The biopsy on your mole came back negative," she said. "It's not

malignant. It was a type of mole called a dysplastic nevi. They're typi-
cally harmless."

It turned out I wouldn't have to revisit the dermatologist after all. I'd
wondered about the results for weeks, secretly hoping there might be
some reason to return to the doctor. Since that brief moment in the sunlight, I would have given anything to cross the street again.

Dr. Fisher closed my chart and settled in her chair and watched me
for a moment.

"Your sixteenth birthday's coming up," she said. "I got a call from your
stepmother, Linda. She and your father were hoping to come see you."

I gazed at her, my eyes wide with disbelief. I didn't know what to say.
Linda felt like some distant aunt I hadn't seen since I was a child. And
I'd buried my dad alongside all the other things I didn't want to re-
member.

"My dad's coming to visit?" I said. "Linda too?"

Dr. Fisher arched an eyebrow. "You look surprised. How do you feel
about seeing them?"

What kind of fucking question is that?

"I'm not sure I can separate everything I'm feeling," I said. "Hurt,
scared, excited. Lots of things."

She crossed her legs and watched me. She seemed satisfied with my
answer. "I also wanted to take a moment to see if you'd given any more
thought to your ninety-six-hour letter."

A ninety-six-hour letter was a written demand to be discharged from
the hospital after a four-day holding period, and it could only be written
by a patient who was sixteen or older. Most of us hadn't turned sixteen,
so writing our "letter" was never an option. But once that day arrived,
our fates were thrust into our own hands. The doctors claimed writing

our letter could serve as evidence that we were a danger to ourselves. We all knew what that meant. It was code for having us committed. Even worse, it was rumored that judges often sent patients to the state hospital.

"No," I said, not quite lying. "I think working on my issues and spending time on chair is helping me."

Dr. Fisher watched me. She knew I had two options. I could cooperate or I could write my letter and try to convince a judge that a sixteen-year-old psychiatric patient didn't need the help of his brilliant, beautiful doctor, who had spent as many years in school as he had alive.

I wasn't stupid. We both knew I wasn't going to write my letter. I wasn't about to gamble between freedom and a state psychiatric hospital.

My sixteenth birthday arrived in early September. By then I'd been on chair restriction for five months. Three of those months had been my summer vacation, and without school to occupy my time I wound up sitting chair as many as ten hours a day. I'd memorized every detail of the new bedroom I shared with Michael. And after spending the rest of my summer vacation studying the shiny new door handles and hospital-grade electrical outlets, they didn't seem very exciting anymore.

It was a weekday morning, just days before my birthday, when Luther appeared in my doorway and said that my dad and Linda had arrived for their visit. My heart sank. I'd been dreading their visit since Dr. Fisher mentioned it the week before. I wondered what they'd think of me, their son, the psychiatric patient.

Luther gestured for me to follow him. I didn't know why. Mom's weekly visits had always been supervised in my bedroom. I slowly got up from my chair and stretched before following him through the security doors and into the new second-floor rotunda. I'd never seen it before. Everything still looked and smelled new. To our right was a small office. He knocked on the door and my dad answered.

"Come on in," he said.

Dad stood up from behind a long conference table and gave me a hug. Luther sat near me, slouching in his chair while he watched us. Linda stayed seated on the far side. Sitting in her lap was a toddler with strawberry blond hair.

"Hi, Banning," Linda said, smiling as always. "We brought you a surprise for your birthday. It's your new brother, Henry."

I went numb and everything fell silent, like a firecracker had gone off in my hand. Linda was still talking but I couldn't seem to hear her. I willed myself to stop caring about them. I wanted them to go away, forever. I wanted them to stop hurting me. The next words I remember Linda saying were "Would you like to hold him?"

I stared at her, smothering whatever love I had left for them. Luther leaned forward in his chair as if something interesting were about to happen. I turned and looked at him, at his small black mustache and beady brown eyes.

They replaced me, I thought.

"We're so lucky to have him in our lives," Linda said. Dad grinned from ear to ear, looking at Henry like he was the son he'd always wanted. He said Adrienne had come home from college just so she could meet him. I don't recall Dad or Linda saying anything else. I only remember Linda handing Henry to me, and I set him in my lap and forced myself to smile while he squirmed and looked at me.

He needs a family more than me. It's not his fault they threw me away.

The visit ended and I returned to my room. For the rest of the afternoon I thought about Henry. I never wanted to resent him; that was more important to me than anything else. I was better than that. I didn't want to be selfish and cruel.

I didn't want to be like my parents.

Tuesdays were family visitation day. My visit with Dad and Linda had been an exception because they lived out of town. The weekly event normally required the use of different bedrooms to accommodate all the parents, which left me to sit in the hallway when our room was occupied. My mom had come to visit earlier in the day, so when the staff escorted Michael and his mom into our room, I shuffled into the hallway and planted myself in my chair.

I was staring at the floor when a bedroom door opened. I turned to see one of the nurses emerge, looking over her shoulder as she guided a bed through the doorway. Then, like a princess on a palanquin, Sonia appeared. She was still strapped to her bed. Her clothing was clean and her hair was wet, and the leather cuffs binding her wrists and ankles had been lined with fresh towels to keep her bedsores from weeping. She craned her neck and grinned at me.

"They let me have a bath," she said.

I held her gaze for a long time, struggling to understand what she'd said. Not the words themselves, but their meaning. How could she be grateful for something so simple? Then I realized a sponge bath was a rare privilege for Sonia. I'd always been allowed to shower in relative privacy, with staff sitting outside the curtain or bathroom, and I'd never been forced to defecate under supervision or ask for help with a tampon or a pad. Somehow, despite being strapped to her bed for months, Sonia managed to find joy in things that I took for granted. I suddenly wondered why I didn't appreciate the little freedom I had left, especially when I didn't have to suffer the same indignities that were part of her everyday life.

Sonia seemed to be having a good day, so the nurse decided to help her with "range of motion" exercises. Joined by another staff member, the two of them moved from one corner of Sonia's bed to the next, making sure to lengthen only one leather strap at a time before relocking its buckle. Then Sonia would lie back and hoist one of her tethered limbs into the air and grimace while she struggled to move the atrophied arm or leg in small circles. After months in restraints, even the slightest amount of exertion left her dripping with sweat.

She was still exercising when Michael and his mom came out of our bedroom and the staff supervising them gestured for me to return to my place inside. But an hour hadn't passed before our room was needed for some parents who had shown up late, so I went back to my spot outside our door.

By then all the other families had left for the night, and the unit was quiet now. Luther sat near Sonia's bed, supervising the four or five of us in the hallway while he wrote in a chart. Sonia glared at the ceiling as if something had happened. I knew her family lived hours away and weren't often able to make the journey to see her. And after an evening of being forced to watch happy family reunions, no one could blame her for being upset.

She was still glaring at the ceiling when Luther broke the silence in the hallway.

"Are you sure you don't want to talk about it, Sonia?"

"Fuck off," she said. "I don't want to talk to you. No one does."

He looked up from his chart. "I think you do."

Sonia kept her eyes fixed on the ceiling. Her hands curled into fists. Luther leaned forward in his chair and lowered his voice, like a man speaking to a frightened child. "Did seeing all the visitors tonight upset you?"

An uneasy tension fell over the hallway. Sonia lifted her head and settled an unblinking gaze on him. She spoke after a long pause.

"No, seriously, Luther. Fuck you."

Luther had shrugged and looked back at the chart in his lap when Sonia lunged for him. Her restraints snapped tight and her shackled hands jolted to a stop, the leather straps trembling as her fingers clawed the air. Luther stood slowly, making sure to stay inches away from her grasping hands.

"You're out of control, Sonia," he said.

She took a deep breath and then pursed her lips and spit in Luther's face.

"Fuck! You! Luther!"

He stepped backward and wiped his mouth and then glanced at his hand. Sonia threw a punch at him and the leather strap fastened to her wrist wrenched her arm backward. She screamed and twisted and then righted her arm, then bent forward and began clawing at her eyes and face. Her fingers snagged in her hair and she grasped a handful of the matted black strands and began tearing them out of her scalp.

"You need to calm down," Luther said.

Sonia stopped and looked at him as if she'd forgotten he was there, her torn black hair still stuck between her sweaty fingers. She leaned back and began trying to pull one of her hands out of the cuff. Slowly at first. Then harder until the leather strap holding it drew tight and began to creak. Then, as her skin and tendons began to stretch, she screamed and her body whipped backward like a rag doll as her hand slipped out of the cuff. She stopped and stared at her hand and smiled before shaking her arm as if to make sure it still worked. A thick band of sores surrounded her wrist, red and angry. Luther took another step backward. Sonia stuck her arm in her mouth and her bared white teeth dug into her skin. She closed her eyes and drew a breath through her nose and then bit down and tore her arm away from her mouth. A long, bloody smear covered her lips. She turned toward Luther standing there awestruck and dazed and spit a mouthful of blood and flesh at him.

Staff poured out of the nurses' station and surrounded her bed. Sonia swung her bleeding arm at them, shrieking and laughing as they tried to pin her down. One of them ran back into the nurses' station and picked up the phone. A moment later a voice spoke over the intercom.

"Dr. Rush to unit H, stat. Dr. Rush to unit H, stat."

Orderlies and staff from the other units began streaming through the front doors, working together to wheel Sonia's bed down the hallway. She bit the inside of her mouth and spit blood at them. Long red streaks spotted their clothing and dripped down the walls. Staff finally got her bed to the entrance to her room, and they pinned her head and limbs to her bed to prevent her from grabbing onto the doorway.

"I'll fucking kill all of you!" she screamed. "Get the fuck away from me!"

They rolled Sonia's bed into her room while the staff waiting inside held down her legs and feet. Luther handed one of them a pillowcase full of restraints from another unit. It looked like a bag full of snakes.

Gloved nurses scurried in and out of her room, holding bloody gauze and bandages. The staff supervising the hallway told all of us to return to our chairs. Whoever had been using our room for a visit was gone now, and Michael was sitting a few doors away. He stared at me as I walked inside, his eyes wide and his mouth barely open.

I remember only sounds for the next hour or two. I remember Sonia shrieking while staff pinned her down to her squeaky bed. Then there were heavy sounds, low and muffled, like two people fighting against a wall. Someone shouted, "Get her arm! Get her arm!" Then the room grew quiet again and I could hear Sonia speaking to someone. Her voice was calm and tired. I closed my eyes and prayed she would stop fighting. Then someone said something and Sonia began shrieking again, and I plugged my ears and closed my eyes and wept until the silence outside felt like the silence inside.

Some time passed. My bedroom was dark and the hallway lights were on when Luther appeared in my doorway. I looked down to see a tray of uneaten food in my lap. I didn't know how it had gotten there. "Unit meeting after dinner," Luther said. He continued down the hallway, repeating the same words to everyone.

Dr. Fisher joined us for the unit meeting. There seemed to be an almost genuine look of concern on her face as she scanned the room.

"It sounds like Sonia's had a difficult day," she said. "I'm sure it's stirred up feelings for everyone. Would anyone like to talk about how they're feeling?"

A few people cried softly. Others spoke for a while. I couldn't listen. I was numb, as if some part of me were still hiding in the quiet place I'd found. I heard a familiar sound from the hallway and turned to see two staff members rolling Sonia's bed into the dayroom. More than a dozen leather restraints had been strapped across her body, all of them covered by a white body net that stretched from her neck to her feet. Underneath it, Sonia lay still, her dark eyes fixed on the ceiling. A thick bandage covered her arm. She looked like a hostage who had been tortured and left tied to a bed in a basement somewhere, her one white pillow a sick gesture of kindness.

"Would you like to say something, Sonia?" Dr. Fisher asked.

The room fell silent. Sonia glanced at her and then closed her eyes and began to cry. Huge tears ran down the sides of her face, her bound hands unable to wipe them away.

Dr. Fisher scanned the room again. Her eyes met mine and I looked away.

"How does it make you feel to see Sonia like this, Banning?"

For months I'd watched the staff provoke Sonia until she bit the inside of her mouth or pissed herself in spite. They restrained and re-restrained her, nudging her ever closer to the same precipice that awaited all of us. Then, after getting her to snap, they paraded her into unit meetings and asked us what it felt like to see her tied spread-eagle to her bed with a dozen leather straps.

"Banning," Dr. Fisher repeated. "What are you feeling?"

How could I possibly describe what I was feeling? I was sixteen years old. I missed my family. I missed going outside. I was tired of therapy. It was hurting me. It was hurting my friends. Every day I witnessed cruelty and violence. How could I explain that? I didn't have the words to express those things. And even if I did, I knew I couldn't admit that I thought the doctors and staff were hurting us. They would throw me in restraints and tell my parents that I was out of control.

Dr. Fisher and the group watched me. I searched for something to say, some safe way to explain everything I was feeling. But when I looked inside myself and tried to understand it all, I saw a huge pit filled with a million things that I couldn't understand or admit, all of them piled up inside me like hundreds of cars that had collided in a foggy tunnel.

I pulled my knees to my chest and hid my face and started crying again.

"I don't know," I whispered. "I just want to go home."

"The group can't hear you, Banning," Dr. Fisher said.

I pushed my forehead against my knees, then closed my eyes and imagined opening them somewhere else, somewhere outside, somewhere far away from the hospital.

"I just want to go home."

6

Without a Scar as Proof

My birthday passed, school began, and autumn arrived, with its longer shadows and darker days. Michael had been out of restraints for a while, and he taught me the ASL alphabet and a few words, mostly profanity, so we could communicate after lights-out without getting caught. A new girl managed to run away during an off-unit appointment. An hour later staff dragged her crying and screaming through the front doors and then tied her to a bed. Sonia still got rushed too, mostly because Luther seemed to hate her for never giving up. But none of it really surprised me anymore. After nine months of being locked inside and sitting in a chair and staring at a wall, everything about the hospital seemed normal now.

The only thing that did surprise me were the new patients. The hospital's expansion had created two new adolescent units, and new faces seemed more common now. Every time they arrived the difference between them and us rattled me. I'd sit in unit meetings and stare at them, fascinated by their opinions and emotions and life. They talked and cried and shook their heads, like caricatures of people, silly and melodramatic. Some of them even laughed for a while. But their laughter never lasted more than a few days. Eventually a soft, gray veil of sadness settled over them, and they became as cold and quiet as the rest of us.

I returned to spending mornings with the teacher who came from my district or working on my assignments in the secure classroom with the rest of the kids. Aside from unit meetings, group therapy, a quick shower, and sleeping, those five hours were my only break from staring at the wall. I'd sit at my desk and rush through my schoolwork while my teacher graded papers. Then I'd open one of my novels and travel with Hemingway to Cuba and Spain to sail and fish and survive hardships that weren't my own.

By early October, Michael and I had been moved to another bedroom, and our new window looked out upon the highway and traffic I'd heard during my trip across the street. And because I was still on chair restriction, the new scene became my only window to the world. I'd rock my chair and gaze out the window at the rush hour traffic, its stream of red and white lights flowing in opposite directions while thousands of people made their way home. I dreamed up stories about some of them. The bitter old teacher counting the days until retirement, and the school janitor just a few cars behind her. Sometimes I wondered if Dr. Fisher was out there too, just another woman stuck in traffic like everyone else.

It was during one of those rush hour daydreams when I heard a polite knock on my open door. I dropped the front legs of my chair to the floor and then looked at the doorway to see Dr. Fisher peering around the corner.

"I need to meet with you in a moment," she said. "I'll be right back." She ducked out of sight and walked away.

Weird. It's kind of late for her to be here.

She came back a moment later, holding my chart. She sat across from me and began scanning some of the pages. She spoke without looking at me.

"I'm sure this will likely come as a surprise," she said.

My heart began to race. *Holy shit. I'm leaving.*

"It's in regard to some recent meetings I've had with your caseworker," she added.

I suppressed my excitement. I didn't want to sound eager to leave.

"My caseworker?" I asked.

"From your father's insurance company. They've decided to accelerate your treatment. Apparently they'd like to see you in a residential program as soon as possible."

"When do they want me to leave?" I said, trying to sound worried. "I'm not sure I'm ready. I still have things I need to work on."

"I agree, so we're going to continue with your current treatment plan, but I'd like to see you start taking day passes away from the unit next week. Soon we'll know more about where you'll be placed and when you'll be leaving."

I felt weightless, like I'd crested a hill in a car and never come down. But as I lay in bed that night and stared at the ceiling, I wondered what it would be like to live in the outside world again.

Maybe it's not the same out there anymore, I thought. *Maybe I'm not the same.*

———

A week later I stood at a rental counter in a bowling alley. A phone on the desk rang while country music played through a speaker overhead. Televisions set to different channels seemed to argue with one another. Bowling balls rumbled into clattering explosions of pins. The manic noise of arcade games filled the background, their chirping and beeping like birdsong in a jungle of sound. Disconnected fragments of different conversations surrounded me. And all of it began reverberating inside my mind, until I wanted to plug my ears and scream.

A voice grew louder, an older woman with a sweet Texas drawl. She repeated herself as if she thought I might not speak English. "What size shoes do you need, hon?"

I knew the words, but they didn't seem to make sense. I imagined closing my eyes and returning to the quiet place inside me that I'd found, but everyone was watching me. I wasn't in the hospital anymore.

The woman spoke again, louder this time. "You'll need shoes if you want to bowl."

"I wear twelves, I think," I said finally.

The woman smiled and grabbed a pair of shoes and set them on the counter.

"Let's head to our lane," Luther said.

I followed him to a slick plastic bench nearby and then kicked off my shoes and slipped on the old pair of rentals. Even through my socks, their worn leather was soft and cool. There was a crash of pins on a nearby lane and someone began shouting, their figure dark and backlit against the bright wooden lanes and white pins. A red strobe on the ceiling began to flash. I wanted to close my eyes; I wanted to turn inward and hide, but my mind insisted on trying to make sense of everything, just like it had for the last nine months.

"Your turn, Banning," Luther said, watching me. Three of my friends sat next to him, wide-eyed and overwhelmed. One of them was the guy with dark brown eyes who had snuck into a girl's bedroom months before. He'd be leaving soon too.

I wandered to the ball return and gazed down at its polished chrome vent as a cool draft of air touched my face. Its soft breeze smelled like the oiled machinery hidden below. I closed my eyes and focused on the air blowing through my eyelashes and hair. It reminded me of being a child, when I used to hang my head out the window of our station wagon and close my eyes and imagine I was flying.

I picked up a ball and then walked toward our lane and eyed my distance from the foul line. The entire bowling alley fell silent. I was alone. It was just me, the pins, and my shot.

I lived in a daze for the next two hours. I remember few details. There seemed to be so much to relearn about the world, and all of it made me feel defective. Music and noise were everywhere. People spoke whenever they wanted. Sometimes they shouted over one another. They laughed and yelled and got angry. And when they spoke to me, it took so much effort to filter out all the surrounding noise that by the time I understood their words they had already moved on to another thought or question. After nine months of living in isolation and evaluating every phrase and action and consequence, my mind had learned to thrive in silence. No one spoke over each other in our tiny world. There were no radios or televisions there. I knew the outside world would be different from the hospital. But for the first time, I realized that my senses didn't.

We played two full games before leaving the chaos of the building. All of us sat quietly in the van while Luther drove us back to the hospital. For weeks I'd assumed my next opportunity to leave the unit would be as incredible as the day I'd walked across the street. But the entire experience had been so overwhelming that I couldn't even tell if I'd enjoyed myself.

Back on my chair, sitting in silence and facing the wall of my room, I was humiliated for feeling at home. I'd adapted to survive the hospital, but there had been no surgery or healing, no stitches or prosthesis. Something else was gone now, and without a scar as proof, no one would ever understand why I didn't work right anymore. Not even me.

Staff-supervised day passes, like our trip to the bowling alley, evolved into unsupervised dinners with my mom. Eventually those weekly dinners evolved into entire Saturdays. But that freedom never extended into my life on the unit. Dr. Fisher and the staff insisted I still needed to sit chair.

"The structure will be good for you," Dr. Fisher told me. "Spending hours away from the hospital can be stressful for anyone. Chair time is for your benefit. Taking you off chair now would only create unnecessary change and stir up more feelings."

She had repeated the same explanation for weeks, and every repetition only made me angrier. The entire idea of chair seemed designed to make me sick. I'd spend hours a day staring at a wall, only to be ripped out of my isolation and thrust into a world filled with people and noise and lights. But I cooperated with her because I knew getting upset would only get me thrown in restraints.

My evenings away from the hospital were pleasantly disorienting. The uniqueness of freedom never got old. Sometimes I'd walk outside the restaurant and wave to Mom through the window and imagine running away just because I could. Our months apart had changed us. And for the first time in years, I thought we might be a family again.

"I love these dinners together," she said one evening. "I've missed being with you."

I looked at her over the top of my menu. I was surprised. Not because of what she'd said but because she meant it.

"I've missed you too, Mom. I worry about you sometimes. I know things were hard for you after Dad left."

She smiled and patted my hand. Her Rolex rattled around her skinny wrist. "Don't worry about me, honey. You just keep talking to Dr. Fisher and Sam and come home soon, okay?"

The following weekend Dr. Fisher announced I'd be going home for my first overnight pass on Thanksgiving. I hid my excitement, but when someone in group asked how I felt, all I managed to say was "I guess I'm kind of scared." When I left the group and returned to my chair, I realized I'd told the truth. I was scared.

Mom drove us to her new condominium for Thanksgiving. It was located in a small rural town called Rockwall. I slept in a new room and bed that Mom said belonged to me, but they didn't feel like mine. I stayed up late and wandered around the neighborhood and stared at the stars. My breath left clouds of mist in the cold air. The silence at night was as black as the sky.

Aunt Martha and Uncle John came out for Thanksgiving. They didn't ask about the hospital. Martha gave me a hug. "I'm sure glad you're coming home," she said. Uncle John watched football and drank beer. He didn't say much to me, he just grumbled at the TV. Mom called Adrienne and we spoke for a few minutes, but I didn't know what to say, so I said "Hi" and "I love you" and then told her I needed to go and gave the phone back to Mom. I loved my sister, but I didn't know her anymore. I went for another walk and Mom drove me back to the hospital.

Throughout December, I sat chair every weekday and went home on weekends. My friends on the unit began to drift away as my departure date drew closer. It's what we'd always done. The moment we knew someone was leaving, we let them go. There was no point in worrying about them anymore. Even Michael and I grew apart. He would be leaving soon too. We stopped signing to one another at night. After lights-out he'd lie on his back and stare at the ceiling, his eyes filled with the same unanswered questions that haunted me.

What am I going to do out there now? Am I even normal anymore?

The week before Christmas, Dr. Fisher explained that my dad's insurance company had agreed to send me to a halfway house in Dallas called Cassidy Place. The facility was located across the street from Timberlawn, one of the largest psychiatric hospitals in Texas.

"We'll be scheduling a time for you to meet with the program manager soon," Dr. Fisher said. "Probably over a dinner pass with your mother next week. Speaking of passes, you've been transitioned through them much faster than usual. How has that been for you?"

"Good, I guess," I said. "But I still don't understand why I have to sit chair if I'm leaving."

"Why do *you* think you're still on chair?"

Jesus. Why does she always ask my questions back at me?

"Because I'm still working on some of my issues," I said. "But everyone in here has issues they need to work on. That's why we're here. Going on pass after staring at a wall is really confusing. I feel weird out there now."

Dr. Fisher arched an eyebrow. "Weird?"

"I just sit there and stare at the wall and think. I can't even *stop* thinking anymore. I've been sitting chair for months now. It's like I'm on chair all the time, even when I'm not. Everything out there feels like it's moving too fast now."

Dr. Fisher nodded without offering an answer or advice. She had done the same thing for months, just staring at me while I talked.

"We should discuss this next week," she said, glancing at her watch. "I apologize, but I have a meeting to attend."

"I'll talk to Sam about it," I said.

Dr. Fisher smiled. I'd meant the comment as an insult.

Michael and his therapist were waiting to use our room when Dr. Fisher left, so I pulled my chair into the hallway to see Sonia tied to her bed. She was drinking ice water from a plastic cup a nurse was holding for her.

"Can I have some of the ice?" Sonia asked, opening her mouth like a baby bird.

The nurse refused.

"Seriously, I can't fucking kill myself on tiny ice cubes," Sonia said. "Just give me some."

The nurse shook her head again.

Sonia managed to slap the cup out of the nurse's hand and knocked the ice all over the floor. She began yelling when the nurse walked away. Staff called a rush a few minutes later, so I stood and waited next to my chair. Then Sonia began slamming her head against the wooden headboard of her bed until a group of orderlies rolled her into her room, where she spent the next hour screaming. Ten minutes later the orderlies walked out of her room and let her scream.

I'd just sat in my chair again when a new girl sitting in the hallway began to cry. She was skinny and had stringy brown hair, and her gray sweatpants and sweatshirt made her look like a prisoner. She sat to my right, covering her face with her hands to hide her tears. She dug her palms into her eyes and began shaking her head as if she were making a wish. *There's no place like home. There's no place like home. There's no place like home.* I remembered when I used to do things like that, when I used to close my eyes and pray that I'd wake up somewhere else. But after eleven months of living in a nightmare, none of it seemed real anymore. My body felt like it had been hollowed out with a knife and all that was left were the broken remains of my emotions rattling around inside me. Even watching Sonia get rushed didn't faze me anymore. I'd stand up and watch the orderlies run past, with their keys jangling and Sonia's screaming and the dull thumping sound of her skull slamming against her headboard, while I just stood there with my back against the wall and a blank look on my face, watching it all unfold as if it were projected on a little screen in my mind, with the nurses and their pillowcases full of restraints, and half the kids in the hallway crying because they still had feelings, because they weren't dead inside, because they were better than me, because they still had a home to return to and parents who loved them.

Mom picked me up that Friday afternoon for one of my overnight passes. We saw each other every weekend now, but Mom still seemed excited that I was coming home soon. We went to dinner that night, like we always did, and I stayed up until she went to bed. Then I bundled up against the cold before kicking my skateboard around the tiered rows of condominiums that scaled the hillside. I'd just sat down to rest when a sliding glass door squeaked open. Two silhouetted figures appeared, a man and a woman. A small flame briefly illuminated their faces as they lit a cigarette and shared a story or a joke. They put their arms around each other and exchanged a kiss. I watched them in the darkness, hating them for their happiness.

What right do you both have to be happy? You stupid fucking people. There are millions of people out there suffering right now.

A horrible pressure grew inside of me. My heart began to race, hard enough I could feel it throbbing against the inside of my shirt. I imagined tearing myself to shreds, ripping the skin from my body until I was nothing but a bloody pile of mutilated flesh. Not because I wanted to feel pain but because I wanted the world to see what I had become, a broken psychiatric patient who had spent the last year of his life watching his friends slowly wither away, until all of us had grown so used to suffering that we didn't know how to be happy anymore.

Then I thought of Sonia, of all the times I'd casually watched her slam her skull into the wooden headboard of her bed. Or all the times she had bitten herself and spit long strings of bloody saliva at the staff. Or the countless hours I'd spent staring at the wall of my room, disconnected from the reality of what my life had become. For nearly a year, I'd insulated myself from the suffering that had permeated my life, until I didn't seem to feel anything at all. And now that I was about to be released from the prison that had become my home, some part of me wanted to lash out at the world for not suffering like my friends and I had suffered.

So instead of skating home or enjoying my freedom, I just stood there in the darkness that night, hating those two strangers for being happier than me. I stood and slammed my board to the ground. Then I recalled Sam telling me to focus on my breathing when I was angry, so I counted every furious breath as I skated toward Mom's new condo. I went to my bedroom and rifled through an old shoebox full of cassettes. Buried at the bottom was my favorite album by Minor Threat. I lifted the cassette out of the box and stared at the spools of tape inside. The last time I'd listened to it was a year before. It hadn't been rewound. I imagined pressing play and magically restarting the life that had been taken from me.

I thought of the first time I'd heard Minor Threat, when I was fourteen years old. It was difficult to relate to that person now, the innocent teenager before the hospital, lost and lonely and looking for a direction. I remembered him. And although I had been sad and confused at the time, I liked the kid who had been trying to find his way through it all. But I wasn't that person anymore. The sense of purpose that had once led me to music and skateboarding had been replaced by a hospital and bitterness and rage.

I pulled on my headphones and watched the spools of tape as I pressed play. The music roared to life, but the kid I remembered didn't awaken.

Two days a week, from Friday night to Sunday afternoon, I lived a normal life. Mom would pick me up and we would drive to Rockwall and spend the weekend together. Sometimes we went to breakfast or a movie and I'd see a familiar face and say something like "Have a good day" or "See you later." Then the person would smile in return and say something similar back to me. The outside world and its people seemed so perfect. Our waitress in her yellow dress and bright red lipstick. The leaves of a tree shivering in the breeze. Even the Texas sunset. All of it appeared so new and beautiful that it seemed surreal now.

The other five days a week, from Sunday evening until my next pass on Friday, I was a psychiatric patient living among the same two dozen people. I knew every nuance of their faces and every article of clothing they owned. Luther's pleated khaki pants and black shoes. One patient's collection of ZZ Top shirts. Another girl's half dozen pairs of sweatpants and bulky cotton socks, all of them painted in the washed-out and shadowless fluorescent lighting that served as our sun. Even our meals were predictable and boring.

But our Sunday night unit meetings were different, when those of us allowed to leave the unit came back and talked about our experience. I remembered listening to those lucky few people when I was new to the unit. Now the new people listened to me.

"Do you think you'll miss the hospital?" a girl once asked me.

She was younger than most of us, maybe fourteen. She sat cross-legged in a huge sweatshirt with a teddy bear on the front.

Everyone watched me while I considered what to say. Weeks before, I'd admitted that I was afraid to leave, and since then I'd spent hours talking to both Sam and Dr. Fisher about it. But no one had ever asked me if I'd miss the unit.

"Yeah," I said finally. "I think I will miss this place."

The girl's eyes grew wide and she sank into her sweatshirt. I remembered feeling the same way when people used to say they would miss the unit. But it was the truth. I knew every detail of our tiny world, from its orange hospital-grade electrical outlets to the number of steps to the nurses' station. I knew our entire selection of small plastic bowls of breakfast cereal and the name of every staff member. I knew which days they worked and the clothes they wore. I'd memorized every detail of the pastel wall in front of my chair. I hated everything about the hospital, but it was the closest thing I had to a home.

Cassidy Place, the halfway house that Dr. Fisher had mentioned, turned out to be a run-down apartment building bordered on all sides by small red lava rocks. The brittle stones spilled over the curb beside the patio and into the parking lot, where they mingled with thousands of old cigarette butts. White plastic patio furniture pockmarked with brown burns stood testament to the generations of smokers who had lived in the halfway house.

"What about school?" I asked Steve, the manager and head of staff, as he finished our tour.

"You'll be attending Skyline, the local high school. And since you don't have a driver's license, you'll probably be taking DART," he said, referring to the Dallas Area Rapid Transit. "The bus stop's just at the top of the drive, across the street."

"What about groceries and shopping?" Mom asked.

"The house receives a monthly stipend for groceries," he said. "All the kids work out the shopping list and budgeting. Then we make a weekly trip to the store. You'll also be responsible for your own cooking, cleaning, budgeting, and laundry."

"What time's lights-out?" I asked.

Steve smiled. "We don't come turn off your lights for you. Life here's about learning to be independent. There's a curfew of nine on weekdays and midnight on weekends, but as long as you're inside, you can go to bed as late as you want. Of course, you're sharing a room, so your roommate might have something to say if you're staying up all night."

The possibility of living anywhere other than the hospital suddenly sounded amazing.

"So what do you think?" Steve asked.

My smile answered before I could. "This is awesome."

Mom looked down at one of the cigarette butts and gently kicked it, as if to make sure it was dead. "Are they allowed to smoke?"

"They're adults," Steve said with a shrug. "I can't stop 'em."

By the end of the interview, I was ready to pack my things and move in. It wasn't until Mom and I left, as I sat in the car and stared out the passenger window, that I heard the same thought that had haunted me for weeks.

I'm different now. I don't even know if I can live out here anymore.

My final two weeks on the unit began with Dr. Fisher telling me I'd been accepted to Cassidy Place. My interview with Steve had gone well and the anticipated vacancy at the house had opened. My discharge date was scheduled for mid-January.

"I can't believe I'm leaving the day before you," Michael signed to me from his bed that night.

I sat up in bed and listened for staff patrolling the hallway.

"Cassidy's cool," I whispered. "Where are you going?"

"Not sure, but I'll miss you, brother."

"I'll miss you too, buddy," I said.

I'd miss everyone from the hospital, whether we had grown close or not. I'd spent the last year of my life watching all of us stare through the warped lenses of our own suffering. Disallowed any privacy or affection, we found solace in glances and whispers and tapping on the walls, all to avoid being punished for being normal teenagers. We had all been re-shaped by the isolation and cruelty of our home. We had been torn apart and reassembled by experiences that would forever connect us. We were a family now, a family that no one outside the hospital would ever understand. And Michael was my closest relative, my brother. He'd spent a portion of our friendship tied to a bed or a wheelchair while I sat in a chair facing a wall. Our only private conversations had been through whispers or rudimentary sign language at night. We'd never even shaken hands. But after helping each other survive a year of fear and pain, I knew we would always be brothers.

Monday, January 18, 1988, began like most of my previous 353 days. The only difference was Michael's empty bed. His farewell party the day before had seemed more like a funeral. Our entire group spent half an hour saying goodbye under the supervision of staff until his mother arrived. Then Michael tipped his head in a teary-eyed salute as two staff members escorted him off the unit. Everyone had begun walking back to their rooms when I turned to see him smile and wave to me through the wire-reinforced windows.

I looked over at his bare bed and its green plastic mattress.

I wonder where he is now.

I got dressed and ready for the day and then sat and gazed out the window, wondering what life would be like as an ex–psychiatric patient. I was rocking my chair back and forth when Luther leaned around the corner of the doorway. It was the first and last time he didn't correct me.

"Time to pack your things, Banning. Your mom just arrived."

I'll never miss you, asshole.

I stood and pushed my chair against the wall and patted its back. Its wooden frame and blue upholstery seemed like old friends now. I packed my two drawers of clothing, walked to the dayroom, and then stood near the doors while everyone said goodbye. Sean, a new patient who had gotten rushed his first week, lay strapped to his bed in the hallway near Sonia's. Together they looked like a matching pair of psychiatric Barbie and Ken dolls. Sonia worked her fingertips around the edge of her body net and waved to me.

"Well, I guess this is it," I said.

"Remember, no shaking hands or hugs," Luther told me.

I looked around at the faces of my friends who wouldn't be going home that night. The unit was the eighth place I'd ever lived and where I'd turned sixteen. It was the first home I'd shared with people who weren't my family or relatives.

Luther stepped around me and unlocked the first pair of doors. I picked up my bag before following him into the elevator-sized security chamber until the doors clicked and locked behind us. I caught a glimpse of Mom through one of the narrow windows as she waited outside in the rotunda. Luther pushed open one of the outer doors and held it for me.

"Good luck, Banning."

I paused and looked at him. It was my last chance to say something hurtful.

He'll win if you turn into him.

"Yeah. Thanks, Luther," I said.

I stepped into the rotunda and Mom gave me a hug.

"Let's go celebrate," she said. "We don't need to be at the halfway house for a couple of hours."

She strolled toward the elevator and pressed the call button while I turned to look at the unit one last time. Through the windows, I could see Sonia and Sean tied to their beds in the hallway. Sean craned his head and grinned at me.

"You okay, honey?" Mom asked.

I didn't know how to answer her. I didn't know if I was okay. I knew I felt weaker and more fragile now. And while I was sure I would eventually be happy to have left, I didn't feel it that night. In fact, I didn't seem to feel anything at all. I just stood there, thinking back through the countless hours I'd spent imagining the day I'd finally escape the hospital, how I'd say goodbye and then walk out the doors and everything would go back to normal, like none of it had ever happened. But as I stood there staring at Sonia and Sean, I knew I would never be normal again, not after months of studying my friends and the staff in hopes of convincing them that I was ready to leave. Not after all the days I'd stared at the wall of my room, until my mind grew so hypervigilant that

I could barely survive a trip to a bowling alley. That evening, as I gazed at my two friends strapped to their beds in the hallway, I knew something was profoundly wrong with me, and the only people who would ever understand were my friends on the other side of those doors. So instead of celebrating that I was free, or cursing the hospital that had wrecked my life, I quietly stood next to my mom as a sickening wave of loneliness and fear crept through my body. I was alone now, and there was no one I could turn to for help anymore. And I wasn't sure there ever would be.

7

We're All Running
from Something

Mom treated me to dinner and then dropped me off at the halfway house. Steve was waiting for me when I stepped inside. I set my bags on the floor and almost sat down before realizing I never wanted to sit in another chair again.

"You ready to go in and meet everyone?" he said.

Steve pushed open the pair of doors that connected his office to the living room. Two girls sitting on a nearby sofa looked up from a conversation. A guy lounging on the floor kept his eyes fixed on a Megadeth video on MTV. A few people wandered around the kitchen, unpacking groceries and getting ready for dinner.

Steve called everyone to join us in the living room. There were about a dozen of us, although some kids were still at work. One by one we introduced ourselves and shared a bit about our backgrounds. Everyone laughed and joked. Steve gave a few people high fives. He seemed more like one of the group than a staff member. After taking my bags to my bedroom, I joined a small group of my new housemates outside.

"Let's head over to the graveyard," one of the guys said. His dark hair and gaunt face flickered to life in the light of his chrome Zippo lighter. He took a drag of his cigarette and then stuffed the lighter back into his black leather jacket.

A short girl standing next to me threw a wad of paper at him. "It's too cold, Pete! Are you kidding?"

"Who fuckin' cares?" he said. "We always take new folks to the grave-yard. Don't be a fucking pussy, Jessica."

We bundled up against the cold and started up the driveway toward Samuell Boulevard, then ran across the street and followed the sidewalk on the far side. The dim lights of a large facility glowed in the distance behind a row of tall oak trees.

"Is that Timberlawn?" I asked.

Jessica ran up next to me. Her frizzy hair puffed out around the edges of her beanie.

"Yeah, that's where the *actual* psych wards are," she said. "I came from there. A few of us did."

Our group cut through an enormous graveyard and walked a quarter of a mile through rows of twilit grave markers and headstones. Some-times we'd stop to look at someone's favorite epitaph or statue, each word and figure illuminated in the sheltered golden flame of Pete's lighter. The cemetery was beautiful in the darkness. I paused and let everyone walk ahead so I could have a moment alone. Tears filled my eyes in the si-lence among the graves. Even after three months of spending weekends at home, it was still difficult to believe that I was free. I stood there for a while, staring at the bare limbs of the trees against the night sky, their silhouetted branches reaching into the heavens, like skinny arms worshipping the moon and stars above.

I caught up to the group as they stopped at the back of the graveyard. A few of the kids leaned against an old wooden fence and lit cigarettes. In the distance, about a hundred yards away, a bright image danced on the screen of a drive-in movie theater.

"Oooh! It's *The Shining*! Yay!" someone shouted.

Jack Nicholson's grinning face filled the enormous screen.

"I love *The Shining*," I said.

Pete flicked open his lighter and lit another cigarette. "Oh, man, you're gonna fit right in."

We settled near the fence and watched the rest of the movie. I sat in the grass at the base of one of the gravestones before leaning back to stare at the sky.

"Want a cigarette, Banning?" someone asked.

"Nah, I don't smoke. Thanks though."

"You mean you don't smoke *yet*," Pete said.

Everyone laughed.

"How long were you in the hospital?" Jessica asked me.

I hesitated. "About a year."

No one flinched. No one laughed. No one got up to leave. Whatever reaction I'd expected never arrived. Then it occurred to me that everyone there could relate. Ever since my trip to the bowling alley, I'd been afraid to leave the hospital, partly because I worried what people would think of me. But beginning in the graveyard that night, and throughout the weeks that followed, I came to understand why I'd been sent to Cassidy Place. The outside world wasn't my home anymore. I had been sent away to live with others like me, kids who lived in a strange land on the outskirts of the real world, like the Island of Misfit Toys. We had schools and jobs, but no home. We had no family, but we had one another. The halfway house wasn't meant to reintroduce us to the real world. It was designed to introduce us to a new one.

Cassidy Place was home to about fifteen kids. All of them were older than me and either attended community college or went to work. My roommate was rarely around. My few sightings of him were limited to seeing his curly brown hair sprouting out from under his covers or the back of his shirt when he left for the day. Life in the house was quiet and simple, and I spent most of my time there alone.

My high school served more than three thousand kids. I'd never been around so many people. There was a convenient but overwhelming anonymity in getting lost in a crowd. Reading and studying at school seemed impossible. People were always talking or chewing gum or clicking their pens. The outside world and its noise seemed louder now. The few friends I made never asked questions about where I lived. A pretty girl in my art class liked me. I liked her too, but I never asked her out. I didn't know how.

Where would I take her? I thought. *What would I tell her?* "Hey, Anna. *Let's go hang out in the graveyard behind the halfway house where I live and sit in the dark and watch* The Shining."

But aside from the stress and strangeness of school, I loved my new home. I'd been entrusted with my own fate for the first time in my life, and I was only sixteen years old. If we blew our budget or didn't plan properly, we'd be low on food and have to fend for ourselves. If I didn't wake up on time, no one came to check on me. I'd miss the bus and have to deal with the consequences. I managed my own bus fare, rides to school, laundry, meals, and countless other things. I enjoyed directing my own life, and I learned more about being responsible for my own happiness in those first three months than I ever had in the hospital.

The house was quiet on weekend mornings when I woke up early to go skating. Sometimes Mom would pick me up and we'd spend a couple of days together, but I usually whiled away my weekends by skateboarding around downtown Dallas or the enormous empty fairgrounds of Fair Park. I spent all week in class daydreaming of racing around those open, sunlit plains of concrete where I could blast music in my headphones and be alone. Nothing else mattered to me. Being free and skating seemed like enough now.

But my memories of the hospital and the friends I'd left behind still haunted me. It was a Saturday morning in March when I grabbed my board and bolted out the front door of the house into the sunlight and clear sky of spring. Once I passed the minefield of lava rocks in the parking lot, I jumped on my board and kicked my way up the drive toward the bus stop, my gateway to freedom.

I stood there in the sunlight, staring at the tombstones and small gate that marked the familiar entrance to the Grove Hill Memorial Home, the graveyard that served as our late-night playground and theater. Then I looked to my left, toward the entrance of Timberlawn, the neighboring psychiatric facility. I'd seen the building nearly every day, but for the first time I realized how ashamed it made me feel.

A vast green sea of well-kept grass surrounded most of the enormous estate, its surface dotted by lush trees and cool, dark shade. Assembled among the trees were long rectangular buildings lined with rows of darkened windows that made the property look like some secret government complex. A nearby parking lot marked the beginning of a driveway that led to a creepy plantation-style house. Next to it, not far from the bus stop where I stood, a white sign displayed the words "Timberlawn Psychiatric Center."

Every morning throughout those months in the house, whether I was going to school or out to skate, I'd lean against the metal pole that marked the bus stop and gaze at Timberlawn, my face burning with guilt and shame. I knew there were people locked inside, some of them probably tied to beds or confined to chairs, gazing out their windows and imagining what it was like to be that guy waiting at the bus stop. And there I was, standing in the sunlight, a few hundred feet away, staring back at them, wondering why I was free to do what I wanted when they were locked inside. Sometimes I'd fix my eyes on a window and picture Sonia and my other friends, all of them still imprisoned in the hospital in my mind, doomed to never leave the place that lived and breathed inside me now.

I wish you were here, I thought. *I'm sorry I'm free and you're not, but I'm thinking of you.*

School ended, summer began, and the house grew even more quiet, since most of the kids worked during summer vacation. I didn't see them often, but they felt something like a family to me. Week after week throughout the summer, we'd cook dinner together and sit on the patio and eat and then walk to the back of the cemetery and watch whatever film was playing at the drive-in movie theater. I'd lie in the grass and stare at the sky through the trees while my friends passed cigarettes to one another.

"Your mom put you in a hospital because you gave away your skateboard?" one of the girls asked me.

"Yeah, and because I said everyone would be happier without me around."

A few kids laughed. "Then every fucking teenager would be locked in a psych ward."

"Do you still talk to your parents?" she asked.

"I still talk to my mom. I haven't talked to my dad in . . ." I thought of him and Linda bringing Henry to the hospital. "I guess it's been almost a year."

Pete sat against a nearby gravestone, lighting another cigarette.

"How can you guys smoke so much?" I asked. "It's no mystery that it kills people. And it's fucking expensive."

"I like smoking," Pete said. "Not to mention, it's better than the shit I used to do."

Pete never took offense. He was only a year or two older than me, but he seemed more mature. He was calm and cool. I envied him. He and a lot of the others in the house talked about NA and AA like they were part of a family. They made mistakes and screwed up. It was just a part of life. There was never any judgment.

"So you've never even smoked weed?" Pete asked.

I shook my head. "No way. I was too fucking scared. My teacher in elementary school used to talk to us about drugs. They had this little poster at the front of the classroom with pictures of pills and syringes. I used to sit there and stare at it. It scared the hell out of me."

"We had the same poster and talks in our classroom," Pete said. "Didn't do shit for me."

I shrugged. "Guess I was too afraid."

Pete flicked the ash off his cigarette. "Sure, maybe you were scared. Or maybe you've just got common fuckin' sense. We've all got issues, man. All of us. I don't care who you are. Show me someone who doesn't smoke weed or snort a line, and I'll show you someone who's eatin' or drinkin' too much." He pinched the stub of his cigarette and squinted as he took a final drag.

"We're all running from something," he said. "But it'll just keep fuckin' up your life if you don't turn around and deal with it."

Weeks later our house manager, Steve, told me he had talked to my dad's insurance company and negotiated my departure date for the end of June. "Looks like you'll be going home soon," he said. Mom was ecstatic. I wasn't. I loved the halfway house. For months I'd cooked my own meals and done my own laundry and gone skating on weekends. My grades had been average, but I'd passed. And even though I didn't often see my housemates, they were my family now. They had been through the system. They were safe. They were like me.

My last meeting with Sam was just a few weeks later. Mom had decided it would be too expensive to keep seeing him and too long a drive from Rockwall. Dressed in his traditional shiny suit, bolo, and cowboy boots, he sat with me in my bedroom while I stared out the open window and listened to the highway. Ever since I'd left the hospital, I'd started feeling anxious when I looked at people while I spoke, but Sam didn't seem to mind my looking away. Sometimes I'd talk about Sonia or sitting chair or never going outside. But no matter what I told him about my time on the unit, I never admitted that I was angry. After a year of watching the staff and doctors restrain my friends, I'd learned to tolerate my anger. Instead, I kept it to myself and pushed it down and breathed it away, worrying over it like a rock in my shoe. I liked Sam, but he was responsible for having me signed into the hospital. When I was there, he was the only person I could trust. But I was free now. I wasn't about to tell him that I was angry now that I was free.

"I'll miss seeing you," I said. "I've known you a long time. You're like a friend to me."

"I hope I *am* a friend," he said.

"You are. You've helped me a lot."

"How?" he said, curious.

"I'm not sure how to explain it. It's like I can concentrate on my thoughts and feelings now. I'll always remember when you had me listen to things when I was in the hospital, when you had me share stories about being outside. That was the only time I felt like I wasn't locked up anymore. Everything seemed to just go away."

Everything. I'd said the word a thousand times, using it as a substitute for all the things I didn't want to remember. But that day, projected in my mind like an image on a wall, I saw Sonia ripping out her hair and scratching her face and her white teeth digging into her arm, and her long, bloody strings of saliva running down the wall next to me. I heard her struggling in Pete's room next door, the buckles of her restraints rattling on the rails of her bed. Then she began to scream, a long, piercing shriek that seemed to come from somewhere inside me, the same place where I'd buried my rage just a few months before.

I tried to speak. My mouth was open. Sam leaned forward in his chair. He was waiting for me to say something, but I couldn't tell him what was happening.

He'll put me back in the hospital.

A breath forced its way into me. My heart was pounding.

Stop thinking about Sonia. Slow down. Focus on something else. Listen to the highway.

I was turning to look at the highway when I heard a long screeching sound followed by a crash. Sam looked out the window over my shoulder. A cloud of white-blue smoke trailed a car careening toward the side of the highway. Another car rolled across the lanes at an awkward angle before coming to a stop in the grass.

"I should call the police," Sam said. He stepped into the hallway to use the phone.

I stared at the accident, imagining that my memories had somehow caused it. A few other vehicles pulled over to the side of the highway and several people got out of them. No one seemed injured. Sam walked back into the room a moment later.

"Everything all right?" he asked.

"Yeah, I guess. I think so."

"It looked like you were about to say something when it happened."

"No, it's okay," I said.

"Heck of a way to wrap up our last session. I don't mind talking for a few more minutes."

I shook my head. "I need to pack anyway."

"Well, Banning, you're going to do well," Sam said, extending his hand. "You've come a long way. You have a lot to be proud of."

I conjured a smile and shook Sam's hand while everything I wanted to say knotted up inside me. I wanted to tell him about my flashback before the accident. I wanted to admit that I'd miss him, but it all seemed too late.

I watched from my window as Sam walked to his car. We had met nearly every week for more than two years. He was one of the only people who had known me before the hospital, back when I was a different person, not fragile and damaged. He cared about my music and asked about my friends. He introduced me to Hemingway. He listened to me talk about my dad and all the times we'd gone hiking and sailing together, and how much I loved the outdoors, and how afraid I was to leave the hospital even though I'd hated being there. Sometimes I thought Sam might have betrayed me, that he was like all the other doctors who pretended to care so they could just get their paycheck and go home. But after months of him coming to see me, I'd started to wonder if he had regretted putting me in the hospital and his way of making it up to me was to help me survive. I knew I'd miss seeing him. But as I watched him drive away, I couldn't help but wonder if he had really been my friend.

8

I'm an Attorney

I was sixteen when I moved to Rockwall that summer. The high school was tiny compared with my old school, with its one parking lot filled with pickup trucks decorated with gun racks and Mötley Crüe stickers. Teenagers laughed in the hallways, threw parties, and went to football games, but it all felt as foreign to me as my first night in the hospital.

The art and band buildings behind the school became my new shelter, and in them I built friendships with the others who came to hide. One of my friends had an absent father. Another's dad was a Vietnam vet who hoarded weapons. The first girl I dated ritually cut herself with a set of razors she kept hidden in her underwear drawer.

These are the kind of friends I want. They make sense to me.

Mom went back to working all the time and helped me buy a car. I got a job at a grocery store and then quit and got another at a car wash. Every weekend I'd drive to downtown Dallas and go skating, just like I had in the halfway house, but it didn't feel the same anymore. Finally, after saving enough money to buy a drum set, I joined a band with a friend of mine from English class. His brother threw me out a week later because I couldn't play as well as their previous drummer.

The next day I took my drums home and directed my frustration into dissecting songs by bands like Black Flag, Descendents, and Bad Religion. There was a strange peace in that place, buried in the intensity of the music blasting through my headphones. Eventually, as my body learned to drum, my mind relinquished control and fell quiet. No thoughts or words or memories appeared in my mind when I played the drums. The outside world and its infuriating noise went away. The ear-bleeding music and its rhythm obliterated everything.

I practiced throughout the winter of 1990, committing hours a day to playing along to my favorite songs while I watched Kuwait's oil fields burn on TV. By then the Gulf War had become something like a reality show.

One afternoon, while I was rifling through my cardboard box full of albums in search of a new challenge, I stumbled across *My War* by Black Flag. The cover's boxing glove, knife, and creepy face reminded me of living with Mom before the hospital. I thought of Sam asking me about it when I first met him. The memory seemed like another lifetime.

I placed the record on the turntable and put on my headphones and then sat behind my kit as the first song began to play.

The opening guitar line began its demented meandering while the high hat and kick drum pulsed in fury. Then, as the bass ascended and every instrument paused, something inside me snapped. A superheated rage came screaming out of me. I closed my eyes and started slamming my fists into the drums as hatred and bitterness wrenched my body. My hands began to burn and I opened my eyes to see I'd split open nearly all my knuckles. I stood and kicked my drums into the wall and screamed until my voice was nothing but a thin rasping sound that tasted like blood. Then I noticed the music had stopped. My chest heaved with deep, angry breaths. I had pulled off my headphones and the stereo lay on its side on the floor, the turntable still spinning and the record a few feet away. The only sound I remember was the faint ringing of cymbals.

My kit lay scattered around the room. The white head of my snare drum was smeared with blood. For a moment I wondered what had happened, as if someone had broken into my room and destroyed everything. Then I looked at my hands, and the blood dripping from my fingers, and my feet standing on the gray carpet of my bedroom floor. Then I thought of Sonia, and all the times she had bitten herself or ripped out her hair, and I realized I was just like her now, filled with so much rage and shame that the only thing I wanted to destroy was me.

The noise and laughter of high school filled me with a seething hatred for most everyone, especially myself. Most people knew me as the creative guy who hung out in the art building and wore pajamas and combat boots to school. But hidden behind my facade was a tortured introvert who spent most of my senior year fantasizing about publicly committing suicide. I reveled in daydreams of shooting myself in the school hallway or hanging above the varnished wooden floors of the gym. I wanted more than to end my own suffering; I wanted to destroy everyone's happiness because I'd never been given my share. So I turned to drumming as my outlet, and I clung to it through my senior year like the controls of a doomed airplane.

I didn't hate everything about high school, though. After a year of "therapy" that seemed more like solitary confinement, something as simple as sitting in the back of the art building and doing my homework felt special. I'd prop open the door and study in the sunlight, then a cool breeze would drift across my arms and I'd begin to cry in happiness. Moments that seemed small and insignificant before the hospital brought tears to my eyes now. It was confusing to feel so ashamed and angry about that year of my life, only to realize that it had given me something very special. I saw beauty in things I had never noticed before. The smell of wet grass and concrete after a storm. The warm Texas evenings and the murmur of the cicadas. The way the wind cooled the sweat on my face when I went skating at night. The worst year of my life had transformed the natural world into something so beautiful that it seemed surreal now.

My friends and those moments carried me through my senior year until my graduation in 1990. Mom was elated despite my barely passing GPA. I took a few art classes at a local community college after getting a job at a nursery, where I could be outside and away from people. Mom and I got home from work around the same time every evening, and we'd talk in the kitchen while we microwaved our dinners before saying good night to eat alone in our rooms. Our days together didn't feel like vacations anymore. Now we were just trying to survive.

"See you in the morning, honey," she'd say.

"Yeah. Good night, Mom," I'd answer.

I spent most of my free time skating around downtown Dallas or playing my drums. Girlfriends evolved into friends with benefits who drifted away because I was afraid of commitment. Then I left the nursery for a better-paying job, only to quit that job months later because I had no ambition.

———

It was a cloudy October weekend when I decided to drive to Bill's, a dirty, disorganized record store in Dallas that was a mecca for music lovers all over Texas. I'd just gotten out of my car when I noticed two guys walking toward me. Both of them wore old T-shirts and cutoff shorts and looked slightly out of place. The younger of the two had long, curly hair that made him look like Weird Al Yankovic.

"We're playing a show," he said, running up to me. "Take a flyer."

"What's the name of your band?" I asked.

"Government Flu."

Jesus, that's a Dead Kennedys song. That's like naming your band Stairway to Heaven.

"I'm Zach," he said. "This is my brother, Doni."

Doni nodded a greeting. He had long brown hair and steely blue eyes.

"We're playing a show at Slipped Disk. You should come out," Zach said.

"Where are you guys from?"

"Sherman," said Doni. It was almost an apology.

We stood in the parking lot and talked for a few minutes. I made a point of mentioning that I was a drummer, so Zach wrote their phone number on the back of one of the flyers before saying we should jam sometime.

They seem like nice guys, I thought as I walked into the store. *Maybe I can convince them to give me a shot at drumming.*

We spoke on the phone several times that week. Zach would set the phone by his amplifier and play his favorite songs. He was only seventeen, but he was a phenomenal guitarist and strung together long, beautiful lines by Jimi Hendrix and Eric Clapton. Doni was studying music in college and was an outstanding bassist.

I knew I'd met two amazing musicians, but I figured I'd be able to keep up with them if we played only punk rock. Eager to prove myself, I offered to drive to Sherman and play a few songs with them. I packed my drums in my car after work that Friday before telling my mom I'd be back on Sunday.

"I'm going to Sherman to try and start a band," I told her.

"Honey, that drumming thing's just a phase," she said. "Please drive safely though, okay? That's a long way to go."

I stayed the weekend with Doni and Zach and their parents in their small two-bedroom apartment. The three of us listened to music all night, rewinding cassettes and lifting needles to replay our favorite songs. But as fun as it was to build a friendship with two genuinely nice guys, my most poignant memory of the weekend was meeting their parents.

The Blairs were unlike any parents I had ever met. Their tiny apartment was filled with faded pictures of when they had met in the sixties, with their hippie haircuts and suede fringe vests. They cooked me dinner and welcomed me into their home. They didn't badger Doni or Zach. They didn't insult them or tell them that playing music was just a phase. Doni and Zach's mom and dad seemed to have complete faith in their talent and ability. There was no doubt or skepticism in their voices, as if they knew with absolute certainty that their unconditional love and support would ensure the happiness and success of their two sons.

"So the boys tell me you live with your mom in Rockwall," Mr. Blair said, tucking a napkin under his beard. He looked at me over a pair of tinted glasses that reminded me of John Lennon.

"Yeah," I said. "I moved there a couple of years ago."

Mrs. Blair appeared from the kitchen, holding a dish of casserole. "But you're from California, right?"

"Born and raised," I said.

"Did you move out here with your mom?" she asked.

I'd briefly mentioned the hospital and halfway house to Doni and Zach, but I never offered details. I hoped they hadn't told their parents.

"Yeah, my dad and stepmom still live there," I said. I almost mentioned my sister, Adrienne, but I didn't know where she lived now, so I awkwardly began inspecting a pair of ceramic salt and pepper shakers that looked like owls.

"Well, you're always welcome here," Mr. Blair said. "We'd love to have you over for dinner anytime."

There was kindness and compassion in his voice, a subtle acknowledgment that whatever my family or the world thought of me didn't apply in their home.

By the end of the weekend, Doni, Zach, and I had formed a band. We took turns driving to and from Sherman to stay the weekend and rehearse. The three of us began brainstorming names for our group, but we never found one that seemed to fit. Then I stumbled across a dictionary I'd taken from my high school the year before. I closed my eyes and opened it to a random page and then planted my finger before looking at the word underneath. Hagfish. We all agreed there was a stupid catchiness to the word that people would remember. Mr. Blair loved the name and drew us a mascot. It was a cartoon fish with an ugly woman's face.

I didn't like the crowds or noise, but I loved playing onstage alongside my friends. Every song was a discussion. Every note and measure expressed emotions that nothing else could. I'd sit behind my kit in some shitty little venue and let my rage come pouring out of me, shaping it into a barely controlled rhythm that Doni and Zach learned to follow. People cheered and shouted and sang along while I demolished one pair of drumsticks after another. An hour later, my ears ringing and body dripping with sweat, I'd move my kit off the stage and then wander outside to pick the wood chips out of the hair on my arms and chest.

Anger wasn't my enemy when I was drumming. It was my fuel.

The last time I saw Mr. Blair was just days before he died. He'd been diagnosed with late-stage colon cancer, and he hadn't responded to the treatment. I went to visit him with Doni and Zach and their mom. All of us, including Mr. Blair, seemed to understand the gravity of the moment. He had lost a lot of weight and looked frail and unhealthy. I made an excuse to leave the room so they could have some time alone. But as I turned to leave, Mr. Blair spoke to me.

"Come here for a sec, Banning."

I walked over and stood beside him while he elevated the back of his hospital bed. A tube from an IV had been taped to his sallow, emaciated arm. He looked at me and smiled.

"I know your dad's not really around," he said. "So why don't you just call me Dad."

Tears filled my eyes. I struggled to speak. "Thanks, Dad."

"You're a good kid," Mr. Blair said. "Don't let anyone tell you otherwise."

He took my hand and gave it a gentle squeeze. There was so much said in that single gesture. I tried to speak but nothing left my mouth, and I didn't have time to say all the things that I wanted. My mind was so crowded with thoughts and feelings, I didn't know what to say.

My words sounded clumsy and stupid. "Love you, Dad."

"I love you too, son," he said.

After Mr. Blair's funeral, Doni and Zach's commitment to music changed. What had once been a hobby became the tireless pursuit of a dream their dad had always known they could accomplish. The love they shared for their parents, and their talent and hard work, seemed to strengthen them, all during a time when I was struggling to hold my life together.

Doni and Zach had ambition and goals for the future.

My only goal was to survive what the hospital had done to me.

My twentieth birthday was three weeks after Mr. Blair's death. By the time it arrived, Doni and Zach had purchased a van and new amplifiers, and committed nearly every free moment to rehearsing or promoting the band. I left Rockwall and moved into a tiny apartment in Dallas so I could be closer to Deep Ellum and Lower Greenville, the heart of the local music scene. I loved drumming and playing shows, but being a successful musician required socializing, and I hated crowds. The shouted fragments of conversations and constant noise were overwhelming. I'd pace the sidewalk outside humid bars until I needed to get my drums on-stage. Then I'd brace myself and run inside and set up my kit while I drowned in a sea of noisy, sweaty, smiling people. I stopped songs to yell at crowds and mock the audience. I left shows early instead of supporting fellow bands. Doni and Zach eventually threw me out, before forgiving me a few weeks later. Then, when I started lashing out at them, they stopped inviting me to rehearsals. This time, they didn't even bother kicking me out. They simply found a new drummer and vanished.

I was crushed. I'd been abandoned again. But as Hagfish grew in popularity, I came to accept that Doni and Zach had found their calling, and that their throwing me out wasn't their fault. It was mine.

"I love drumming," I mused to a friend. "But maybe I'm meant to do something else. I couldn't stand the crowds anyway."

"What are you going to do now?" she asked.

"I don't know," I said. "I've never really thought about it."

Without a band to keep me busy, I picked up shifts at my retail job at a local mall called the Galleria. The shopping center was an enormous glass monstrosity filled with shops and restaurants and an ice-skating rink. The noise inside was horrendous. Music and voices carried from one end of the mall to the other. But after living in isolation for so long, I discovered it was the perfect place to study people. Since the day I'd left the halfway house, I'd felt like an impostor, a shadow wandering the land of the living, studying people to make sense of things as trivial as eye contact and small talk. Did the Cowboys win or lose? Is it supposed to rain this weekend? I didn't like my job, and I hated the mall, but after months of practicing basic social skills, I began to feel more like a person than an android pretending to be a human being.

Mom moved back into the room above Martha and John's garage that summer to save money. Their house was close to my apartment, so once a week she would treat me to dinner at one of our favorite local restaurants. Dressed in one of the designer business suits she always wore to the travel agency where she worked, she'd get out of her beat-up Toyota and wave to me through the window. I loved my mom, probably because she was the only family I had left. But every time I saw her dressed up, all I saw was a sad old lady trying to convince herself that she wasn't depressed.

Each week we asked each other the same questions and shared the same answers.

"How's work?"

"Fine."

"Are you seeing anyone?"

"No."

"You look tired."

"I am."

It wasn't until months later, during one of our dinners, that Mom first mentioned the hospital. I thought she was going to cry. I'd never seen her feel remorse for anything. I froze and stared at my plate and didn't say anything.

"I'm so sorry I put you in there, honey. I didn't know what else to do. I was so scared."

"It's okay," I said. "It's not your fault."

"Every time I left the unit after coming to see you, the doctors would sit down with all the parents and tell us if we took you out early that we'd come home and find you dead." Tears filled Mom's eyes. "I would die, honey. I would die. I couldn't live without you. You're my little boy."

It wasn't the first time Mom had mentioned my committing suicide since I'd left the hospital. She never referred to it directly. She only talked about how horrible it would be "if something happened to me." We both knew what she meant. I didn't know what to say. I wasn't exactly suicidal, especially now that I was free. I just didn't want *this* life; I wanted a better one, so I went on hoping that my better life might arrive someday.

"I just want you to be happy," she said, wiping her eyes. "It makes me so sad to see you lonely. I'd love for you to meet a nice girl and get married."

I turned back to my dinner. "I'm twenty-one, Mom."

"But all you do is work and go home and sleep," she said. "You used to go outside and play in the dirt in the backyard."

"When I was in second grade or something."

I tried to enjoy the rest of our meal, but Mom kept talking about how wonderful our lives were when I was a kid, as if she had forgotten alienating Adrienne and bribing me to steal Dad's bills and then leaving me at the airport, but I never mentioned any of it. I just wanted to forget about my past now.

"Can we take the rest to go?" I asked. "I can eat it for dinner at work tomorrow."

I called in sick the next day so I could enjoy the bright November morning. After making a pot of coffee and opening all the windows, I sat on the floor to sketch a picture out of an old magazine. I was eating lunch in front of the TV when the phone rang.

A deep voice spoke in a slow Texas drawl. "May I speak with Banning Lyon, please?"

"This is him."

"Mr. Lyon, were you held in a psychiatric facility a few years ago?"

My heart began to race.

"Why?" I asked.

"Banning, my name is Parks W. Bell. I'm representin' a friend of yours who mentioned your name. I'm an attorney."

"Who are you representing?"

"Well, Mr. Lyon, that's attorney-client privilege," the voice said. "However, there's a gentleman who'd like to ask ya a few questions about your time in the hospital. He's an associate of mine named Robert Andrews. Ya give'm a call and tell'm Parks W. Bell sent ya. Ya got somethin' to write his number down?"

I wrote the phone number on a piece of paper and then dialed it when he hung up. The line rang for a few seconds before a friendly voice answered.

"Andrews and Clarke."

"I'm calling for Robert Andrews. My name's Banning Lyon. Parks W. Bell just called me."

"This is Robert," he said. "I'm glad you called, Banning."

"Parks said you're representing someone I know?"

"Do you remember Kevin Mardason?"

A dozen memories flashed through my mind. I recalled Kevin strapped to his wheelchair and the ridiculous voices of his fictional alter egos. I could still picture him singing and laughing in the hallway with Sonia, and his messy Elvis-style hair.

"Yeah," I said, smiling. "I remember Kevin."

Mr. Andrews explained that he was representing Kevin and wanted to ask me some questions about the hospital.

"If you've talked to Kevin, then you probably know everything already," I said. "He was there a lot longer than me."

"I'd still like to hear your side of things, Banning. My office is in the Team Bank building in downtown Fort Worth. Would you be able to make it out here soon?"

I scribbled down the directions to his office and hung up, a thousand questions racing through my mind. I'd only spoken to a handful of people about the hospital, and the idea of talking to a total stranger about it, let alone an attorney, filled me with a sickening fear.

I left work early the next day. It was after six o'clock when I found the building. I signed in with the security guard before taking the elevator to the twelfth floor. The doors slid open to reveal a small, dimly lit lobby. "Andrews & Clarke" was printed in plain black letters on a frosted-glass door. I stepped inside to find a row of chairs and a sad-looking plant sitting across from an unoccupied receptionist's desk. When no one appeared, I called out.

Robert shouted from somewhere in the office. "I'm back here. Down the hallway to your left."

I wandered past a conference room and into a small office. Piles of manila folders and boxes covered the floor. Pens and binder clips were scattered everywhere. A huge window on the far side of the room looked out over downtown Fort Worth. In front of the window, a jolly-looking man sat half hidden behind a stack of documents on a desk. Hanging on the wall next to him was a small wooden plaque that read "Kill all the lawyers."

"Hi, Mr. Andrews," I said.

He groaned. "No mister, please. Just call me Robert. I'm only thirty-nine."

He stood and introduced himself and then reached out and shook my hand. He was short and had messy salt-and-pepper hair that was just a little too long, like a Franciscan monk who'd become an attorney.

"Sorry to make you drive so far," he said. "I hope it wasn't an inconvenience."

"It's cool. I didn't have anything to do except watch *Star Trek*."

He almost jumped out of his chair. "I love *Star Trek*!"

I didn't know what I'd expected, but I was surprised to like him so quickly. He spent the next few minutes raving about his favorite *Star Trek* episodes before rummaging through his desk for a yellow legal pad to take notes.

"Before we get started," he said. "I want to remind you that I'm representing Kevin in a case against the hospital. I'm not your attorney, but if we both agree that you're here for a consultation, then everything we talk about will be protected by attorney-client privilege. Do you understand?"

"Sure, I guess, but I don't really have any money," I said.

"Don't worry about that. I just want to talk to you about your stay in the hospital. If there comes a time when I represent you, well . . . we'll cross that bridge when we get there." He leaned back in his chair. "Before we talk about the case, do you mind if I ask you a few questions about yourself?"

"Go ahead."

"Tell me about your warts," he said.

I stared at him, confused for a moment. I didn't know how to answer the question. "Well, I had a few warts when I was in the hospital, but they froze those when I had the mole on my chest removed. I had a big one on the ball of my foot too, but I was just a kid."

Robert grinned. "I'm sorry, I should've made myself clear. Not *actual* warts. Your shortcomings. Do you drink? Do drugs? Have a criminal record?"

"No, I don't drink or do drugs. I'm straight edge," I said, pointing at the small X-shaped tattoo on my hand.

"Then what would you say your biggest shortcoming is?"

I answered without thinking. "I hate people who wear an unearned smile. And I hate the sound of laughter."

Something like compassion filled Robert's eyes.

"What about Dr. Fisher?" he asked.

I shrugged. "I don't know."

"Do you hate her?"

"No. I usually like women more than guys."

Robert wrote that down.

"Have you ever heard of a thirty-minute chair?" he asked.

A familiar image of my old room's textured pastel wall flickered through my mind.

"Yeah, I know what chair is," I said.

"Indefinite chair?"

I nodded.

"Restraints?" he asked.

The word sounded strange outside the hospital. No one out here was supposed to know it.

I nodded again.

"Do you think they use restraints and chair therapy in other hospitals?"

"I don't know." I shrugged again. "I guess every hospital does stuff like that."

"Why do you think you were kept in the hospital, Banning?"

"Because I gave away my skateboard."

"But why do you think you were *kept* in the hospital?" He paused as if he'd set a gun on the desk.

"Just my opinion?"

Robert smiled. "Just your opinion."

"Insurance. No one really left because they got better," I said. "Most people left because their insurance ran out."

"Do you think the hospital charged your dad's insurance company for chair therapy?"

"For sitting in a chair and facing a wall? I don't know. I don't see why insurance would pay for that. I just sat there."

"What if I told you that NME, National Medical Enterprises, the company that owned the facility where you were held, paid kickbacks to people to refer kids to hospitals like yours?"

Robert's words awakened a memory from a time I'd long forgotten, when I was skating down the sidewalk after school and my counselor spoke to me from her car.

I want to talk to you about your skateboard.

Robert continued. "What if I also told you that some diagnoses received more insurance money than others. For example, a hospital might receive only five thousand dollars from an insurance company to treat someone suffering from alcoholism. But if that same patient suffers from depression, the hospital might get ten thousand dollars or more, just by giving that person a different diagnosis."

I recalled my last week on unit B before being sent to the adolescent long-term unit. I thought of Dr. Anderson and his rodent-like teeth and his telling me that I suffered from severe depression.

Robert spoke again, reciting the words as if he had said them hundreds of times. "Banning, are you aware that Senator Mike Moncrief and Texas attorney general Dan Morales were both involved in having NME investigated for paying kickbacks for patients?"

I don't know how long I sat there staring out the window behind Robert. All I remember are questions.

What else will I learn if I join the lawsuit?

What will happen if we lose?

What if I really needed to be in the hospital?

What if they try to put me back in?

9

Lookin' for Patients in
All the Wrong Places

National Medical Enterprises had already agreed to pay nine million dollars to the state of Texas as a penalty for aggressive marketing and admission practices, including paying for patient referrals. But as Robert frequently reminded me, those fines weren't guilty pleas and did nothing to help those of us who had spent months or years locked in the hospital.

I joined the lawsuit a week later, on December 5, 1992. Days after I agreed to become a plaintiff, Robert called me on speakerphone. I could hear someone speaking to him in the background when I answered.

"There's someone who'd like to talk to you, Banning," Robert said.

Kevin's cheerful voice was as endearing as I remembered. We reminisced about the hospital for a few minutes before we ran out of things to say. Then I realized I didn't really know Kevin. We had lived together for months, but we had never spoken outside the hospital. It seemed strange to feel so close to someone I hardly knew.

"Kevin's story was featured in the *Houston Chronicle* this morning," Robert said. "They've been covering the lawsuit for a while. I'm sure they'll want to talk to you soon too." The telephone clattered as Robert picked up the handset and took me off speakerphone. "I need to run to a hearing, but I'll give you a call later this week. Get ready for things to take off."

"Hey, wait." I said. "I don't want to just sit back and be a plaintiff. I don't know what I can do to help, but I can make copies or lick stamps or something. This isn't just about money for me. It's about something else."

"I understand, Banning. It is for me too." He paused for a moment. I could almost hear him smiling. "How about coming out and meeting Julie and the kids this week? It'd give me a chance to explain the statute of limitations in your case."

I made the hour-long drive to Fort Worth the next afternoon. When I arrived, Robert's brown Volvo was parked next to a Mercedes station wagon in front of a cookie-cutter suburban home. He was still wearing his suit from work when he answered the door.

"Hi, Ban," he said. "Come on in."

I'd been given so many nicknames throughout the years that I'd lost count. Bingo. Bandit. Banjo. Bananarama. But Robert calling me Ban seemed to fit, and it made me happy to know he felt comfortable enough to say it.

The house was in the same disarray as his office. I weaved through an obstacle course of children's toys to find countless books scattered around the dining room table. There were Bibles printed in Hebrew lying next to boxes of comics. Stacked against the wall were dozens of romance novels with frayed spines, bodice rippers with bare-chested men and busty women on the covers. Each of them looked like they had been read three times. None of the men looked remotely like Robert. Then I noticed a beloved book from my childhood. It was a first-edition *Dungeon Master's Guide.*

"You play D&D?" I asked.

"Julie and I have played Dungeons & Dragons for years, ever since we were in seminary. David, our oldest, plays with us now."

"You went to seminary?" I asked.

"I studied to become a minister before I went to law school."

I followed Robert into the kitchen, where he introduced me to his family. His wife, Julie, had short strawberry blond hair and a friendly Texas accent. She looked like a cheerful high school choir teacher, wearing a Christmas sweatshirt even though it was January. She stepped away from the stove and gave me a hug and then sat me down at the table.

"David, can you say hello to our guest, please?" she said.

A young boy with black hair trimmed in a Dutch-style bowl cut sat across from me. He nodded politely.

"Hello," he said.

Their two sons, Paul and David, were both adopted. David looked to be about five years old, but he spoke like an adult. Paul sat wiggling in a high chair beside him while Robert said grace.

It had been more than two years since I'd eaten a meal with a family, back when Doni and Zach's parents used to invite me over on weekends. I hadn't had a meal with my own parents and sister in ten years. Being a stranger at a table had always been difficult. I'd sit quietly and eat my food and laugh when everyone else did, as if I were pretending to be part of the family. But Robert and Julie and their kids somehow managed to make me feel as if I'd eaten with them a thousand times before.

Throughout dinner, David blurted out random facts about space and the periodic table of elements. Julie talked about meeting Robert while she was studying music in college. Now she was a piano teacher and taught at the local seminary. And Robert—I couldn't have described Robert to anyone. Before dessert was on the table, he managed to explain how comic books inspired him to study theology and become an ordained minister before going to law school. I barely understood half of what he'd said.

Julie offered to clean the table after dinner so Robert and I could talk more about the lawsuit. She gave him a friendly hug and a peck on the cheek and then shooed us into the living room.

"I know I've already mentioned the statute of limitations," he said. "But I wanted to go into some detail, since it's our biggest hurdle. The law states there's a given length of time you have to sue someone, depending on the crime. For example, there's no statute of limitations for murder or tax evasion, but you only have five years to sue someone for insurance fraud.

"However, it's possible to argue that someone should be able to file a lawsuit later if a crime is discovered. So, using the earlier example, if insurance fraud is uncovered years after it was committed, then a judge might extend that five-year statute of limitations so people could file new lawsuits."

Robert went on to explain that the most crucial portion of my case was convincing a judge to extend that statute of limitations.

"You had faith in the people operating the hospital, and they exploited it," he said. "It wasn't until the government investigated NME that you could've possibly known they were paying bribes for patients."

"But what if the doctors were right?" I asked. "What if I did need to be there?"

Robert turned to me and said nothing. I thought of Dr. Fisher appraising me during one of our sessions, but something in Robert's eyes was different.

"Banning, if you did need to be there, and I don't believe that you needed inpatient care, what you received was not therapy. All of you were hostages being held for insurance money. To NME, you kids were just golden geese laying golden eggs."

Six years had passed since I'd left the hospital, six years of isolation and loneliness and secrecy. I'd spent countless hours of my life obscuring my past, pretending the hospital hadn't ruined me, that I wasn't some defective ex–psychiatric patient. But as I sat there with Robert, staring at his dining room table covered in D&D manuals and theology textbooks, I realized that he didn't care if I was wounded. He saw something else in me, something valuable, something worth saving.

By the end of January, the lawsuit had taken over my life, and the once unfamiliar drive to Fort Worth turned into an almost daily ritual. Robert's office became something like a sanctuary, a place where legal petitions and document boxes and the stale odor of warm coffee came to represent the possibility of a new life.

February brought the conclusion of our hearings on the statute of limitations. The judge ruled to extend my statute's deadline and allowed my case to proceed. Robert was ecstatic. He called me after leaving the hearing to tell me the good news.

"This is it, Ban. We've won the most important battle of the war. NME is probably shitting its pants right now. They never thought this would happen, and now we're going to fight them in the papers."

Robert called every journalist willing to listen to him. Sometimes he'd introduce me to one of them over the phone before asking me to share something about my story. I'd never spoken openly about the hospital, about my memories of sitting chair or the things I'd witnessed. It wasn't until Robert introduced me to Jonathan Eig, a writer from *The Dallas Morning News*, that I realized people didn't think I was broken. They thought the hospital was broken.

Jonathan was waiting at Robert's office when I arrived. He looked to be in his late twenties, but all that remained of his downy hair had retreated to the top of his head. He followed us to the conference room and sat with his back to the window, taking notes while Robert sat next to me and listened.

"I hate people," I said. "I hate the world. I hate everything because of what they did to me. I just wish I had some kind of time machine and I could go back to being fifteen."

Jonathan scribbled in his notebook. "And you were initially told you'd be there for two weeks?"

"Yeah, for an evaluation," I said.

Robert leaned forward. "Banning was there a total of three hundred and fifty-three days before being sent to a halfway house."

"What did that wind up costing the insurance company?" Jonathan asked him.

"Banning's father's insurance ultimately paid around a hundred and sixty-six thousand dollars."

Jonathan flipped a page and kept writing. "And you said you think this is just the beginning. Any idea how many people you might wind up representing?"

"It's impossible to predict," Robert said. "We have about eighteen right now, and we're working on nearly twenty more. I'd say it'll reach the hundreds."

We talked for another half hour or so, but mostly I listened and stared out the window while Robert and Jonathan discussed insurance, legislation, and policy change, things that sounded bigger and more important than a handful of broken teenagers. The economics of what had happened to us never mattered to me. I didn't care whether the insurance companies had sued National Medical Enterprises, or that the government was investigating them. When I thought about the hospital, all I saw were images of a girl tied to a bed, and the wall of my room, and the faces of the people who had hurt us.

Eventually Jonathan got up to leave. He collected his things and followed Robert out of the conference room, and I trailed behind them, still lost in my thoughts. I was staring at the floor when Jonathan walked over and shook my hand.

"Thanks for sharing your story," he said. "People need to hear it."

The Dallas Morning News printed Jonathan's article on April 26, 1993. By the end of the week, the entire lawsuit had changed. Phones rang constantly. Boxes of documents piled up. A couple of weeks later I got home from work to find a message from Robert on my answering machine. His voice was quiet and serious.

"The attorneys for NME sent over a couple of boxes of discovery today," he said. "There's a few things I'd like you to see."

I drove to Fort Worth that weekend. When I arrived, the office was quieter than usual. Robert called my name from the conference room and I walked in to find a television on a wheeled cart peering over a mountain of papers and boxes. Robert stood half hidden in the corner, digging through the pile like a man stuck in a snowdrift.

"We're going to need a storage facility soon," he said.

He made his way over to the television and pushed a tape into the VCR.

"I found this video in one of the boxes," he said. "It was made shortly before you were signed in to the hospital."

I moved a stack of documents out of one of the chairs and sat down when the television cut to a scene of a cowboy riding a horse. Rolling golden hills filled the background behind him. A tinny guitar began to play the tune "Looking for Love in All the Wrong Places." The whole thing seemed like a bad karaoke video.

What the hell does this have to do with the hospital?

The camera cut to a close-up of the cowboy just as he began singing, but all the words of the song had been changed. Then the familiar chorus began.

"No more looking for patients in all the wrong places . . ."

The cowboy continued singing the parody, twisting the lyrics into a detailed explanation of how to target kids with good insurance in hopes of locking them up for at least six months. The cowboy grinned stupidly while he rode his horse. He seemed pleased with himself. Robert stood next to the television, watching me while I stared at the screen. The cowboy sang another verse and chorus before riding into the sunset, then the video trailed off into static.

"This was used to target patients like you, Ban. Kids from broken homes with good insurance policies. They knew divorced parents asked fewer questions." Robert turned off the TV. "If a jury sees this video, it's over."

I couldn't tell where my pain began and my anger ended. I wanted to put my fist through the television. I'd grown up thinking of parodies as something funny, like "Weird Al" Yankovic songs, not videos about predatory mental health care. The whole thing seemed so cruel. I opened my mouth to ask something, only to close it after realizing there was nothing to understand. I'd lost a year of my life because my divorced parents had good insurance. I almost said I was angry, but the words sounded stupid before they came out, so I didn't say anything.

Robert began digging through one of the boxes on the floor. He had his back to me. I was looking out the conference room windows when I heard a sound I'd long forgotten, the bright metallic jingling of buckles.

"I'm sorry to show these to you," Robert said, "but I'm curious if they're familiar."

He pulled a long leather strap out of the box. The cuff of a restraint dangled from one end. There was a look of innocent curiosity on Robert's face. The restraints were covered in scribblings. I could see Sonia's initials and the letters *FTW*. My mind replayed a memory of Sonia speaking to Dr. Fisher during a unit meeting.

"It means 'Fuck the world,'" Sonia said.

I stood up. The conference room suddenly seemed long and narrow. A soft static filled my ears, like the sound of the ocean in a conch shell. Robert looked like he was miles away. His mouth was moving but I couldn't hear him. I reached out to him, but my arms didn't move. My body wasn't mine anymore. I shuffled toward him, disoriented, as if I were wading through a river. Sonia seemed stranded in my peripheral vision, tied to a bed in a room somewhere nearby, here but not here. She was looking at me and screaming and tearing fistfuls of wiry black hair out of her scalp. I tried to yell but nothing happened. My mouth didn't even open.

Robert called my name. His voice seemed muted and faraway. He reached out and put his hands on my shoulders. His arms looked ten feet long.

"You're not in the hospital anymore, Ban. You're here. You're safe."

I opened my mouth to speak, but nothing came out.

"I'm sorry," he said. "I thought since you hadn't been in restraints, it'd be safe to show those to you. I just wondered if you'd recognize them."

I stumbled back to my chair and sat down. My shirt was soaked with sweat.

"I didn't think I'd ever see those again," I said. "They were Sonia's."

Robert sat next to me. We were quiet for a long time.

"I want you to remember what I'm about to tell you," he said finally. "You didn't deserve what happened to you in that place. None of you did. Some of you kids truly needed help, but what you received wasn't therapy. It was abuse."

All the pain I'd stored inside me began spilling out. I buried my face in my hands and let go, sinking into the chair as I curled into a ball and wept. After a while, Robert set his hand on my shoulder.

"This lawsuit's going to be harder for you than it is for me," he said. "It could take two or three years and require months of trials in a courtroom. You're going to have to retell your story over and over, including memories you may have forgotten or blocked out."

I wiped my face on my knees and looked at him. "I don't know if I can do this," I said.

"Ban, if you can make it this far after everything you've been through, I know you can do this." He smiled and squeezed my shoulder. "And this time you're not alone. This time you have me."

Until that moment, I'd never known what it was like to believe in someone, to feel with absolute certainty that someone would never give up on me. It wasn't the first time Robert had said he would always be there for me. He had probably said something similar at least a dozen times before. But for some reason, maybe because I was curled up and crying in a chair in his office, his words that day finally came to rest inside me, as if they had found their way through all the doubt and fear and pain that my parents and the hospital had left behind. Robert sat beside me for a long time that day. I don't remember if he said anything else. His promise was the only thing I'd ever wanted to hear.

10

Life as You Know It Is Over

By midsummer the corporation that owned and operated the hospital had shut down or sold many of its psychiatric facilities. The media attention had hurt them and they were under pressure to divest of anything associated with mental health care. Within a month, Robert had gotten permission to walk through the units where many of us had been held, so he invited me and Kevin and a handful of others to join him.

I refused at first. I knew it made no sense to be afraid of the place. It was closed. But the idea of seeing it again filled me with terror. For years I had avoided the stretch of highway that passed the building, even if it meant driving twice as far.

"They'll be tearing down those units soon," Robert said. "This'll be your last chance to walk out of that place on your own terms. I'll be there with you. Some of the other kids will too. I won't let anything happen to you while we're there. I promise."

A week later our little group of ex–psychiatric patients met at the hospital. It was early afternoon. The building looked the same as the day I left, with its pale brick walls and screened windows. I stopped my car at the far end of the parking lot and sat in silence while I stared at the hospital. Robert was standing out front with a few of my friends from the unit. I locked my car and walked toward them, making sure to keep my eyes on the hospital. Everyone greeted me with smiles and hugs and nervous laughter. Robert patted my shoulder to remind me he was there. Then he led our group inside.

We arrived at a pair of double doors, the same ones I had stepped through six years before, when I stood in the sunlight and listened to the sound of the birds and the wind. I stopped at the threshold and looked back at the scene that still lived so vividly in my memory. I remembered the warm concrete through my socks, and the sparrows chattering, and the flag and its halyard snapping in the breeze. The murmur of cars on the highway was still there.

I was turning to follow Robert when I stopped and stared at the hallway. I didn't want to go inside. Robert put his hand on my shoulder. "No one's going to hurt you, Ban. Not with me here."

We stepped into the shaded hallway and crossed the rotunda before making our way through the empty offices and nurses' stations we had never been allowed to see. Every unit looked deserted. Loose papers littered the floor. Most of the furniture had been removed, leaving behind a collection of faded squares and rectangles in the gray commercial carpet.

Over the next half hour, our small group slowly separated as each of us went to revisit an old bedroom or gaze out a familiar window. My first bedroom had been on unit B, but none of my friends had stayed there, so I wandered off by myself.

I paused in frightened reverence outside my old doorway, then I stepped inside to stare at the place where I'd slept six years before. The thin gray carpet lay dusty and bare, and two bright rectangles marked where the beds once stood. Even without the furniture, the room conjured hundreds of memories. The night my appendix almost ruptured. The kind nurse who held my hand on her knees. The nauseating smell of cigarette smoke.

Robert stepped into the room and stood next to me. I felt safer with him there. I started crying. He grabbed me in a tight bear hug. He was so short. I stood there paralyzed, looking down at his scruffy salt-and-pepper hair.

Stand still. He's not going to hurt you. He promised.

Before long Robert let me go. I wiped my eyes and he took a step backward and kept his hands on my shoulders.

"That's the closest to an exorcism I've ever performed," he said.

It seemed a strange thing to say until I remembered he had studied to become a minister. I wiped my eyes and laughed, probably to keep myself from crying again. Robert lowered his head and closed his eyes.

"Lord, remind Banning of his strength and courage. Guide him on this journey of healing, and help him find compassion for himself. The only meaning to be found in this place is for him alone to find, and I pray that you'll help him find it. Bestow your love and guidance upon him, and forever walk alongside him on his quest to find his own answers."

Robert gave me a final hug and we stepped out of the room. We found the rest of the group waiting in the hallway outside, so we all walked together toward the parking lot, down the same corridor I'd walked through when I first went outside and listened to the birds and the highway.

"So what's it like not to be a victim anymore?" Robert asked.

I stopped.

"What the hell does that mean?" I said.

"NME has already made settlement offers. They haven't been good ones, but they're offers. And those offers are going to get better. They know it's inevitable. There's going to come a time, probably soon, when they make an offer worth accepting."

I stood there staring at him, wondering for the first time if he was just another selfish attorney. Robert stepped toward me and I backed away.

"They're never going to admit to any kind of wrongdoing, Ban. A settlement's likely the closest to an admission of guilt all of you will ever receive. It's important for you to accept that, for your own well-being."

"So what am I supposed to do? Just forget what happened here?" I said. "Are you fucking serious? You're telling me I need to just *move on?*"

"Just think about it. I'm not trying to argue with you, and I'm not saying you don't have a right to be angry. You do. But you can't let them keep hurting you. If you want revenge, you need to take the strength that helped you survive this place and use it to find happiness."

"Sure!" I shouted. "I'll just take the money and be healed! Halle-fucking-lujah!"

I stormed to my car without saying goodbye to anyone. By the time I'd shoved my keys in the ignition, I could feel my heart throbbing in my face. I cranked the engine and jammed my car into gear and then stomped on the pedal, swinging a long, screeching arc across the parking lot before slamming on the brakes. I sat there and gazed out the windshield at the two-story, windowed monolith where some part of me still seemed to be trapped. For a moment I wondered why I was still afraid of the place. After all, I was free now. And after meeting Robert and talking to reporters and seeing how horrified they were by what had happened there, I knew that most everything about the hospital was wrong. Even the company that owned the building wanted it torn down. But maybe that's what terrified me about the hospital, that it wasn't a building or a place; it was a symbol of everything wrong with me and my life, a symbol of selfishness and greed, and tearing it down wasn't going to fix everything that had happened to me any more than it would fix the system that kept me and my friends locked inside until our insurance ran out.

I turned twenty-two that September. By the end of the month, the lawsuit's initial flood of discovery and depositions dwindled to a steady stream of obscure legal mail that made no sense to me. So, with only a part-time job and a couple of classes at a local community college to keep me busy, I adopted a dog. Tundra had long white fur and dark eyes and a perpetual grin that made her look like a smiling arctic fox. She was barely six months old. The first time my mom saw her, she thought I'd gotten a stuffed animal.

I still drove to Fort Worth to see Robert, although I was still angry about his saying that I wasn't a victim anymore. I wouldn't have admitted it to anyone, but after years of struggling to protect myself from my family and the hospital, I had no other identity. The idea of being something other than a victim didn't just frighten me; it was impossible to imagine. Surviving was all I'd ever done. Without it, I was nothing.

One afternoon in early October, during one of my visits to the office, Robert asked me to write a short story about the hospital. He sat me down at a desk and handed me a pen and a legal pad and told me to write a few pages about the first thing that came to mind, so I spent the next hour scribbling a story about Luther and Michael and the one time I jumped on my bed. When I handed the pad back to Robert, he skimmed its pages and then stashed it in a drawer.

"What are you going to do with it?" I asked.

"A friend at the *Times* wanted to see what you had to write. He said if it's any good he might consider publishing it."

I shrugged. "Well, it's a piece of shit."

"We'll let him decide," Robert said.

A week later I got home from a morning lab class to find my answering machine at the end of the cassette, which usually meant someone had accidentally left their phone off the hook instead of hanging up. I had pressed the rewind button and then started a pot of coffee and sat with Tundra to listen to the message when the machine clicked to a stop. The tape began to hiss and a woman's voice spoke over some noise in the background.

"Mr. Lyon, this is Connie Chung from CBS News. I read your op-ed in *The New York Times*. I'd love to talk to you. Call me back when you get the message, please."

I looked at Tundra. "Holy shit. I used to have a raging crush on Connie Chung."

The tape kept playing. Reporters. Talk-show hosts. Even someone from *The Oprah Winfrey Show*. All of them had left more than a dozen messages on my answering machine.

Oprah called me. What the fuck's going on? How did they get my number?

Then Robert's perennial reminder resonated in my mind. *Don't talk to the media.*

I called his office and he answered on the first ring. He sounded worried. Phones were ringing in the background.

"Connie Chung just called me," I said. "And Oprah."

"You didn't talk to them, did you? Jesus, I can't keep track of all you kids right now. Can you come out here, Ban? We'll go grab lunch. I've got to get you away from the phone."

I arrived at the office an hour later. Robert grabbed his coat and barked something at his secretary and then drove us to a local burger joint. He hardly spoke during the drive. He just grinned and stared out the window. We had just sat at one of the picnic tables outside when Robert went into a long explanation of how all the media pressure had frightened National Medical Enterprises.

"Your op-ed changed everything," he said.

I set my burger on its greasy wax paper and stared at the table. "But what about all these people calling? What do we do now?"

"Nothing yet. I'm not going to let you call Connie Chung unless NME keeps softballing their offers, but now your op-ed gives us some leverage. Something tells me their offers are about to get a lot better." Robert paused for a moment. "Ban, eventually you're going to get a settlement offer worth considering, and it won't involve a judge or a jury or any kind of plea deal. It won't be an admission of guilt. NME wants to buy your silence."

"Then why don't we take them to court?"

"We can make a difference without them pleading guilty," he said. "I'd love to take them to court, but there's no way to know what'll happen in a trial. I'm almost sure a jury would find them guilty. But juries are unpredictable. And it could take years." Robert pushed his lunch and drink to the side and looked at me. "As your attorney, I think you need to consider any fair settlement offer. But as your friend, I want you to imagine what it would be like to live through another two or three years of this lawsuit only to see a jury find them not guilty."

"But they *are* guilty," I said. "You told me we have a great case."

"We do, but years of legal work isn't free. We'd have to hire more help and the fees would keep piling up. Settling for less might actually mean more money when you consider the cost of another year or two of legal work. Remember, NME has millions of dollars and a team of attorneys on retainer. We can't outlast them."

"But what if they're are still locking up kids?" I said. "What if they're still using restraints? If I don't do something, then *I'll* be responsible. It'll be *my* fault."

Robert grabbed my hand. "Banning, none of this will ever be your fault. Ever. Don't you ever think that. You don't need to take responsibility for what they did to you."

I stared down through the cracks between the boards of the picnic table. A small brown sparrow hopped around looking for crumbs.

"You didn't deserve what happened to you," Robert said. "Do you remember me telling you that? Your parents let you down and NME took advantage of it. Even if you accept a settlement offer, I still want you to remember that what they did was wrong."

I nodded, even though I didn't know what to believe.

"Don't worry," Robert said. "I'll keep reminding you as the years pass. You're not rid of me yet."

———

I never spoke to Oprah or Connie Chung. I never went to court to testify before a judge or jury. No one ever pleaded guilty or admitted to any wrongdoing. Two days after the publication of my op-ed in *The New York Times*, National Medical Enterprises offered to settle our class-action suit for fifteen million dollars.

I was sitting on the floor with Tundra when Robert called to tell me. A wave of joy swept over me. Then relief. Then something like emptiness. Since the beginning of the lawsuit, I'd had friends and a purpose and something to accomplish. Now that it was all over, I suddenly felt like I'd lost more than I'd won.

For months Robert had warned me to have a plan for the settlement, saying on more than one occasion that some of my friends' parents had already asked them for money. He told me to have something ready to say if anyone, even my family, came asking for a loan.

"Write what you want to say on a piece of paper and stick to it," he said, "like a script."

I'd already called two financial advisers and both of them said the same thing: invest the money in stocks if I wanted to be wealthy or purchase a type of annuity called a structured settlement if I wanted to be stable. The choice wasn't difficult. But when I told Robert I was planning to put almost my entire share of the money in the annuity, he sounded shocked.

"What about college or a trust?" he said. "What about traveling?"

I picked up the notes I'd written down and started rattling off some of the benefits, including how the annuity would be tax-free and that it couldn't be claimed as a possession if someone sued me.

"I just want to stop worrying," I said. "I'm only twenty-two. I don't have a family or anything to fall back on. I don't know how to invest it and stocks are unpredictable. I'll waste it if I can get my hands on it."

"I'm proud of you," he said. "I think you might be putting too much away, but it's not my decision to make. Not to mention, it'll give you something to tell anyone who comes asking for money. If you don't have any lying around, then you've got none to give."

I laughed and told him I didn't think that would ever happen.

All he said was "I sure hope you're right."

Later that week I got home to find a message from Robert saying that all the settlement documents would be ready to sign in the morning. I called Mom and told her I had some good news, so she offered to meet me for dinner at one of our favorite restaurants. It wasn't far from my apartment, maybe a mile or two, so I decided to walk.

The restaurant was dark and quiet when I arrived. All the tables and booths were empty. A hostess stood alone at the bar, rolling silverware into black cloth napkins. She glanced over her shoulder and smiled and asked if anyone was joining me. I said my mom was on the way, so she grabbed two sets of silverware and seated me near the front door. It had been propped open to let in the autumn breeze, and a long, golden blade of late-day sunlight streamed through the open door.

I closed my eyes and rested my chin in my hands.

Six years ago I was sitting in a chair facing a wall. Now I'm about to start a new life.

I still had my eyes closed when Mom walked in. She said something and gestured for me to give her a hug before sitting down. We chatted until our waitress arrived and, without looking at the menus, we both ordered chicken potpies. I was folding my napkin in my lap when Mom spoke again.

"How's our lawsuit going?"

Our lawsuit. Robert's warning appeared in my mind. *Friends and family are going to come asking for money.*

"It's over," I said. "They finally made a decent offer. I'm driving to Fort Worth tomorrow to sign the paperwork."

"I bet your *New York Times* article helped, honey. It sure was beautiful."

"It wasn't just that," I said. "It's been hard work for all of us."

I held my glass of water on the table with both hands, staring at it as I ran my thumbs through the condensation. Three words repeated themselves in my mind, like a vintage neon sign. *Please don't ask. Please don't ask. Please don't ask.*

"Have you thought about what you'll do with the money?" Mom asked.

Have something ready to say, I thought. *Like a script.*

"I talked to two financial advisers and they both said the same thing. I should put the money in a structured settlement. It's the only chance I have to do it, since it has to be transferred directly to the annuity company." I took a sip of water and recalled my notes at home. "Over the course of my life, it almost triples what I'm getting. And it's tax-free. I might use a little to go to college or travel, but I won't have much left over."

Mom's face wilted. "Haven't you thought about buying a house?"

I shook my head. "I might get a house someday, but I'm too young now. I don't know what I want. That's why I got the annuity."

"We could get a place together," she said. "I've been looking at houses in McKinney."

Stick to your script. Robert warned you. Don't feel guilty and selfish.

"Mom, this is the best we've ever gotten along. I don't want to ruin this. If we went back to living together, we'd just argue all the time. I want to move forward, not backward."

She brightened her voice. "Then maybe you could help me buy a house?"

"I already told you. I'm not going to have any money left over," I said. "If I keep it, I'll waste it. I'm tired of living from paycheck to paycheck."

"But they're building a lot of new houses out in McKinney and Allen. They're really affordable."

I hung my head. "I've already explained this to you. I'm getting a structured settlement. I can't go back and get it later. This is my only chance."

Mom hardened her voice. "Honey, I'm in debt. The hospital hurt me too. I *deserve* some of that money."

It wasn't the first time my mom had insisted the hospital had hurt her. But after years of dealing with flashbacks and anxiety, I wanted to scream at her for suddenly demanding a share of what amounted to a year of my life.

I shoved myself back in my seat. "Then sue them yourself, Mom. If you really feel that way, then you should do something about it."

She froze and narrowed her eyes. She stared at me for a long time before wrestling her purse out of her lap and standing up. She lowered her voice to a whisper.

"Banning, if you don't help me, I'll make sure you don't get a dime of that money. I'll go to Connie Chung and Oprah and all those people who called you and tell them you won't even help your own mother. I'll tell them you *deserved* to be in that place."

Mom turned and stormed out of the restaurant.

I was still staring at the doorway, hoping she might reappear, when our waitress arrived and set two beautiful chicken potpies on the table.

"My mom left," I said.

The waitress didn't say anything. She just stood there with the tray under her arm and a sad look on her face while tears pooled in my eyes.

"I guess I'll go," I told her. "I'm sorry about this."

I didn't know what else to say. I got up and wandered out of the restaurant and back toward my apartment, sobbing while I followed the sidewalk. Tundra lay asleep on the bed when I got home. I curled up next to her and called Robert. The kindness in his voice made me start crying again.

"Why do I even love my mom?" I said. "She doesn't even love me. She's never loved me. She didn't even want to pick me up at the airport. I wish I could just hate her."

"I'm so sorry," Robert said. "I was hoping she wouldn't do this."

I sat up and wiped my eyes. I was staring out the window when he spoke again, his voice lighter now.

"Why don't you call U-Haul and rent a truck?" he said. "Pack up all your things. Put Tundra in the front seat and drive out here. You can stay with me and Julie and the boys. You can find an apartment out here. We love you. We'd love to have you near us."

"I can't break my lease," I said. "I'll lose my deposit."

Robert burst into laughter. "Banning, you're a millionaire now. Fuck your lease. Go rent a truck, pack your stuff, and drive out here. I'll wait up for you. I don't care what time you arrive; just call me when you're leaving."

"But what about my car?" I asked.

"We'll get it later. It'll be safe at a U-Haul," he said. "I'll drive you back to Dallas to pick it up. If it gets towed, you can buy another one."

I laughed and wiped my runny nose on the back of my hand. "This is it. It's over. The lawsuit's finally over, isn't it?"

I could hear Robert smile over the phone. "Grab a piece of paper and a pen, Ban. I want you to write something down."

I thought he was going to give me the phone number to U-Haul. I reached over the side of my bed and grabbed a yellow legal tablet I'd taken from his office. There was a black Sharpie marker clipped to it. I propped the phone between my cheek and shoulder.

"Write this in big letters and hang it on your wall," he said. "Life as you know it is over."

I tore off a page and then turned it sideways and scrawled the words in thick black lines. Then I hung the paper on the wall next to my door with a single thumbtack.

I passed the note every time I carried a box to the truck that night. Tundra and the note were the last two things to leave my apartment.

It was four in the morning when I finally pulled up in front of Robert and Julie's house. All the lights were out and I wondered if Robert had gone to bed. I climbed out of the truck. Tundra sat up in the front seat, watching me as I walked to the house and tapped on the front door. I was about to go back to the truck and let her out when I heard someone fidgeting with the doorknob.

Robert appeared in the doorway, still wearing his suit. He was missing one shoe and looked half asleep. Behind him, in the darkness, lay a minefield of toys and books. Behind me were all my belongings, my dog, and the strewn-out wreckage of my family and past.

Robert rubbed his eyes and shuffled toward me with his arms wide. I was crying by the time he reached me. Whatever exorcism he had intended for me in the hospital months before came to its conclusion in that minute-long hug. He squeezed tears out of me I'd been holding inside for ten years.

Then, like Robert always did, he kept his hands on my shoulders and took a step back to look at me and smile.

"Welcome home, Ban," he said.

11

Robert Franklin Andrews

I woke the next morning to a house filled with the sounds of a kitchen and cartoons and laughter. Tundra lay asleep on the floor nearby, curled up with her nose tucked under her tail like a white fur shawl. She followed me downstairs, where Paul and David sat giggling in front of the TV. Julie was cooking breakfast and reading one of her romance novels. She handed me a cup of coffee and then sat me down at the table while Robert paced around the house with the phone sandwiched between his shoulder and ear. I was halfway through a stack of pancakes when he pulled up a chair next to me.

"The settlement documents are being sent over to the office," he said. "We'll need to head over there as soon as you're ready."

The office was quiet when we arrived. Robert sat behind his desk and I planted myself across from him. His secretary set a stack of papers in front of me. Colored sticker tabs and bright yellow highlighter decorated most of the settlement agreement.

"Sign and initial each page where it's marked," she said. "Get comfortable. You'll be here awhile."

I thumbed through a few pages. Every phrase looked confusing and dangerous. The names of the doctors and staff dotted the text. Sometimes I'd stop to read a condition or stipulation before giving up and initialing the page and moving on. An hour later I slumped in my chair and stared at the agreement, wondering exactly what I'd signed. Robert pushed a calculator toward me and then handed me a note.

"Enter that number," he said. "That's your share of the settlement before legal fees."

Written on the paper were seven digits beginning with a one. There were two commas.

Holy shit. I am a millionaire.

"Now divide that by three hundred and fifty-three," he added. "Then divide that total by twenty-four. That's how much you were paid for every hour you spent in the hospital."

I stared at the numbers for a long time. For a moment, I was angry or disappointed or some confusing mixture of both. It seemed unbelievable that a year of my life and freedom could amount to something so simple. All my days of sitting chair and eating alone and watching Sonia get rushed. All of it had been reduced to a second-grade math problem. Then I heard Robert's words from our day at the hospital, when he said that my greatest revenge was to find happiness. I hadn't understood his comment at first. But now, as I gazed at the value of those 353 days, something made sense.

Every time I pay rent or buy gas, or get a cup of coffee or dinner for a friend, or if I ever buy a wedding ring or a gift for my kids, I'll be taking pieces of the hospital and turning them into something beautiful.

After eleven months of doubt and fear and hope, I suppose I'd expected the end of the lawsuit to feel more dramatic, that I'd sign a few documents and then walk out of Robert's office a different person. Instead, after staring at those numbers, I realized that all I'd won was an opportunity, and that nothing had really changed. I was still me, only now I had an annuity and a chance at a new life.

By the end of the week, I'd rented an apartment near a private community where Robert and Julie planned on buying a house. I never went to get my car. Mom had helped me buy it years before, so I gave it back to her and bought a Range Rover, my one frivolous purchase to celebrate the end of the lawsuit. Along with my old car, I also gave Mom ten thousand dollars because I felt like a terrible son for not buying her a house. When I called to make sure the wire transfer had gone through, she went on a tirade about my new sister.

"She's already three or four," she said. "Your father and Linda named her Emily. That was going to be your name if you'd been a girl. They didn't even care enough to tell you."

The truth was someone had told me and I'd forgotten. Since the day Dad and Linda brought Henry to the hospital, I'd ignored them or blocked them out. Then I'd see something or hear a name and a memory would rise to the surface. I couldn't recall who had told me about

Emily. I assumed it was probably Dad, but I had no memory of his voice or when he could have told me. As far as I was concerned, I didn't have a family now.

Eventually Mom stopped complaining and thanked me for helping her. She said she loved me and I said, "I love you too."

When we hung up, I knew we wouldn't speak again for a long time. My mom finally had her money, and I finally had her out of my life.

My annuity barely covered my rent and expenses at first, but if I maintained my familiar diet of ramen and peanut butter sandwiches, I didn't have to work. I was never forced to leave my apartment or socialize, and Robert and Julie and the kids became my only connection to the world of people.

I spent weeks aimless and lonely. The lawsuit had given me a sense of purpose. Now I didn't know what to do with my life. There was nothing to overcome. I had no routine and I never wanted to work again. My only ambition was to avoid more hardship. I didn't know anyone in Fort Worth, so I bought a computer and played games for days at a time. Sometimes I'd drive around or go to a coffee shop, hoping to meet a girl, but I didn't know what to say when it happened. One girl asked me where I worked, but when she saw my Range Rover, I wasn't sure know how to explain how an unemployed twenty-two-year-old guy managed to buy an expensive British off-road vehicle that he only drove to the coffee shop.

After that, Robert and Julie started inviting me to church. I disliked going, but I went anyway because I was grateful for their love and kindness. I knew they only wanted me to be happy, but every introduction led to the same questions.

"So where do you work, Banning?"

"What do you do, Banning?"

After a few visits, I found a quiet room on the second floor where I could hide until it was time to go home. It seemed to be the only way to avoid explaining the rabbit hole that had become my life.

It was one of those Sundays when Robert and I stood outside the church while we waited for Julie and the kids. The doors of the chapel opened and a woman peeked out. She looked to be about Robert's age. Her short brown hair and thick glasses made her look like a cheerful church mouse.

"Hi, Sharon," Robert said. "Did you ever meet Banning?"

A smile brightened her face. She stepped out from the chapel and leaned forward to look at me. "Oh yes, I remember you. Banning Lyon."

"I hired Sharon as a consultant during the lawsuit," Robert said. "She's a nurse. She read all your charts."

"I tried to keep my distance from all of you," she confessed. "I wanted to remain objective. I probably read over a hundred of those charts. I read yours more than once." She grinned and shook her head. "Awful stuff. I wanted to throw myself off a bridge after the first weekend of reading."

I couldn't help but laugh. It was easy to like Sharon. There was something endearing about a nurse joking with an ex–psychiatric patient about jumping off a bridge.

We spoke for a few minutes before she hurried off to find her husband. A light mist had started to fall, so Robert and I had stepped back inside when we ran into Sharon's son. He looked a little younger than me, with his mom's curly brown hair and easy smile. Robert introduced him as Nathan.

I remember being tired and talked out and wanting to be alone that day. But the moment Nathan spoke, I felt normal, like I was sitting in the graveyard with my friends from the halfway house. Instead of asking what I did or where I worked, he asked if I played D&D or board games or wanted to hang out with him and his friends. I don't remember what I said. I probably just nodded or started talking about D&D. What I do remember is feeling like I'd met someone important, and that I hoped we'd meet again.

On June 29, 1994, The New York Times reported that National Medical Enterprises, the company that had operated our hospital, had settled a yearslong lawsuit filed by the Justice Department. It turned out that NME had agreed to pay the federal government $362.7 million. It was the largest health care settlement in U.S. history. Peter Alexis, a former executive for NME, pleaded guilty to charges involving bribery and kickbacks. He admitted in court that more than fifty doctors and others had received payments during the time I'd been locked in the hospital.

The news reignited interest in our case and cast a spotlight on a life I wanted to leave behind. Weeks later, several of us from the lawsuit, including Robert, were invited to speak before a congressional committee on health care fraud and abuse. The invitation was an incredible privilege, but I was too tired to keep retelling my story. I hated being the poster boy for psychiatry gone wrong. I also worried about the consequences of appearing because I'd agreed in the settlement not to speak about the case for a while.

"Testifying in front of Congress is usually granted legal immunity," Robert told me. "If there were ever a safe chance to tell your story, this is it."

I wasn't going to change my mind. But no matter how times I told him I didn't want to talk about the hospital anymore, I still felt like I was disappointing him.

"I understand," he said finally. "I'm proud of you for being able to say no."

He reclined his office chair and then stared out the window as a smile crept across his face. "The other day Paul asked me if you were *really* his brother. I think both the boys see you as a brother. Paul can't remember a life without you."

"They *are* like brothers to me," I said. "I hope they know that."

"I wouldn't worry. It's normal to them. It's adults that don't get it."

Robert distracted himself with one of his pipes before settling back in his chair. He drew a few puffs and started picking at something on his desk.

"How would you feel if we wanted to adopt you?" he said.

I felt like I'd been kicked in the stomach. For as long as I could remember, I'd wanted a family more than anything else. Now that I was being offered one, I was terrified. I didn't want to be abandoned again. I sat there and wondered what to say that wouldn't hurt Robert's feelings. No one had ever done so much for me or deserved more, but I didn't want a family, not after everything my parents had done to me. I hated the word. I hated everything associated with it. Holidays. Anniversaries.

Birthdays. Weddings. The word conjured images of sitting alone in the Dallas/Fort Worth airport and praying my parents would come get me. I didn't want another family, not after everything they had done. For a moment I imagined running out of the room and driving home and pretending Robert had never even mentioned it.

"I can only imagine what you're thinking, Ban," Robert said. "But I don't want to replace your family. I just want you to know that we love you, and that we'll always be here for you, no matter what happens. That's what families are supposed to do." He choked up and wiped his eyes. "Julie and I both love you. I'd be proud to call you my son."

I forced a smile and then turned and looked out the window.

"Take your time and think about it," he added. "There's no rush. But if you remember one thing today, please remember that all of us love you, and that we'll *always* be your family, no matter what you decide."

A few days later I dragged myself out of bed and downstairs to start a pot of coffee. I'd stayed up all night playing games and gone to bed after sunrise. Tundra stood in the kitchen, wagging her tail while she waited for breakfast. I was rattling kibble into her metal bowl when the phone rang. It was Robert. He sounded scared.

"Your apartment complex is gated, isn't it?" he asked.

"Yeah, there's a security guard at the gate. Why? What's wrong?"

"The doctors sued us today."

My heart stopped. I leaned on my desk.

"Why?" I asked. "Sued us for what?"

"For libel and defamation, for the newspaper and magazine articles they already released us for in the settlement agreement. They sued Sean, too."

"But they can't," I said. "They already released us for that stuff."

Robert realized he had scared me and softened his voice. "People can sue anyone for anything. That's how our legal system works. They're just lashing out because NME settled with the government. They're afraid for their reputations. The suit's frivolous. It'll get dismissed."

He had said the words in one long run-on sentence, as if he were trying to convince himself of something he didn't really believe. I sat at my desk and stared through the floor.

"So what do we do now?" I asked.

"Don't answer your door if someone knocks. They might try to serve you. When it gets dark tonight, bring Tundra over here and plan on staying for a few days."

I looked into the kitchen to see Tundra smiling at me. Her black eyes seemed to wonder what was going on.

"I'll order pizza," Robert said. "We'll stay up late and play D&D. Try not to worry. This'll all blow over soon."

I was served with the lawsuit later that week. Robert helped me find an attorney, since he was a defendant in the case and couldn't represent me. The initial shock of being sued drifted into months of indecipherable legal mailings and waiting for something to happen, all while I accumulated a legal bill greater than my means to pay it. I stopped leaving my apartment and spent the next few months taking only brief breaths at the surface of my life. It was then that I began hiding from my anxiety and panic in the only place that felt safe, the world inside my computer.

Christmas Eve arrived. It was Robert's birthday. He called the day before to invite me over to the house. I pried myself away from my computer and packed up Tundra and a small bag of clothing. We stayed up late that night and wrapped gifts for the kids. We drank eggnog laced with rum and watched Christmas movies and laughed while my mind oscillated between the same two thoughts.

This is the happiest I've been in a long time.

The doctors are suing me.

Every morning of those days at the house, I woke up to Paul and David jumping on my bed and Julie cooking breakfast. Then I'd stumble downstairs and grab a cup of coffee and sit outside and gaze at the backyard. The morning of Robert's birthday, I sat with a book and managed to read for the first time in weeks. He had given me the novel as a Christmas gift. It was *Time Enough for Love* by Robert Heinlein.

"It's about love and life and family," Robert told me. "It's one of my favorites."

I finished a chapter and folded the book closed and then stared out across the yard at the clear morning sky. White frost powdered the lawn and trees. Robert cracked the door to the patio and the sound of cartoons and the kids' giggling streamed outside. He sat nearby and read a book in the comfortable silence of not needing to talk. Paul peered through the door and then laughed as he darted away.

Maybe this is what family's supposed to be, I thought. *Maybe this is where I belong.*

My adoption required nothing more than going to the courthouse and claiming Robert and Julie as my parents. Our judge was a middle-aged man with dull brown hair that made him look like a senator. Robert knew him. The judge grinned while we stood together at the front of the courtroom and proclaimed ourselves a family.

"Julie and Robert, do you both understand this adoption is permanent and that Banning will be your legal child?" he asked.

They were standing on opposite sides of me, away from each other. Robert looked at me and smiled. Julie took my hand and squeezed it.

"Yes, your honor," they said.

"Banning, do you understand this adoption is permanent, and that Robert and Julie will be your legal parents, regardless of whether they remain married or not?"

My stomach slowly twisted into a knot. I didn't want to be adopted, but I wanted to make Robert happy. I was afraid I'd lose him if I didn't go through with it. In my mind, I was alone. An individual. Disconnected from people. I had been in sixth grade when I last had a family. I was twenty-three now. I hadn't spoken to my dad and Linda since I was in the hospital, and I couldn't remember the last time I'd talked to Adrienne. And my mom was a bitter old woman who cared more about money than happiness. But the adoption seemed so important to Robert. I didn't want to let him down, not after everything he had done for me. Julie seemed uncertain too, although she never mentioned it. She was always kind and loving to me, but there was a distance to her friendliness that made me wonder if she wasn't ready to have another son.

"Yes, your honor," I said finally.

The judge signed the order and congratulated us. Robert led us out of the courtroom. Julie trailed behind with the kids in tow.

"I'll always be your pop, and your father will always be your dad," Robert said. "But I'll be damned if both of us being named Robert wasn't a sign."

The weekend after my adoption, Julie hosted a small get-together to celebrate. I had spent all night playing games on my computer, and I arrived late to find the house filled with guests. Music and happiness flowed through every room like a warm breeze. Julie smiled at me from behind her piano. People I had seen at church hugged me and shook my hand. Robert was introducing me to someone when I recognized Sharon McCoy, the nurse he had hired as a consultant on our lawsuit. I asked about her son from church and Robert gestured toward the back of the house.

"He took over the computer in my study," he said. "Go on back and say hi."

I walked past the living room to find Paul and David goofing off in front of the TV. I picked them up by their ankles and tossed them on the sofa before wandering off to Robert's study. Nathan sat facing the computer with his eyes fixed on a game.

"What are you playing?" I asked him.

He glanced over his shoulder and grinned. "Oh, hey, Banning. It's this new game called *Warcraft*. You pick a team, either orcs or humans, and you build a town and mine gold to upgrade your buildings, but you have to defend it while you try to destroy the other guy's town."

I propped myself on the edge of the desk and listened while he explained the game. I usually avoided people I didn't know well, but something about Nathan made me feel comfortable. Talking to him seemed effortless. Long passages of silence didn't feel awkward or strange. I probably sat there for half an hour, chatting and laughing with him, before I realized how easy it was to be around some people.

There had been a time before the hospital when making friends came naturally to me. I could still recall my mom's stories about how gregarious I was as a child, how I'd come home from kindergarten and say I'd fallen in love with some girl or made a new friend, or the way I'd lean over the back of a booth in a restaurant and smile and wave to a group of strangers.

"You'd just smile and laugh," she would say. "People loved you. You could talk to anyone."

Mom's retelling of those stories changed after the hospital. We would go out to dinner and she would gaze out the window and mourn the once happy child I'd replaced. The boy she remembered haunted me. He was gone now—the hospital had killed him—and Mom's stories seemed to be all that remained of him.

But as I sat in Robert's office that day and watched Nathan play a game, I felt like that kid again, when I used to call my friends on Saturday morning to see if they could ride their bikes or go swimming, back when relationships were simple and easy and I didn't have to explain where I came from or why I didn't work or how I managed to buy a Range Rover.

Weeks after my adoption, Robert asked if I wanted to take a road trip to Arkansas to meet his mother. Robert was one of the worst drivers I had ever known, so when I expressed apprehension at spending hours in a car with him at the wheel, he conceded and let me drive.

"Fine by me," he said, reclining the passenger seat of his new Mercedes. "That'll give me time to read. But I get to pick the music."

We made our way through Little Rock and north across rural Arkansas, where old barns and rusty tractors lay sleeping in fields of tall green grass. Robert lit his pipe and then folded a paperback in one hand and read while we listened to Neil Young. Eventually the highway dwindled to a two-lane road that meandered past small towns with names like Bald Knob, Oil Trough, and Pocahontas. We were somewhere between them when Robert switched CDs and the Who's *Tommy* began to play.

"You know, when I first met you kids, I thought of Tommy," he said, mumbling with his pipe between his teeth.

"Why? He's deaf and blind, isn't he?"

"Tommy was trapped in a prison," he said. "It might have been his own mind, but it was a prison. The album's not just about surviving hardship. It's about finding a way to let hardship make you better. The doctors stole your innocence, just like Tommy. But you found a way to survive and you're stronger because of it. You should be proud of who you've become."

For as long as I could remember, I'd wanted my dad to say the same thing to me.

"Thanks, Pop," I said. "It's nice to know I have at least one dad that's proud of me."

"Please don't ever think your father wouldn't be proud of you. A lot of years have passed. He's probably as afraid to reach out as you are."

Robert leaned back against the headrest and turned to look out the window. He was quiet for a long time.

"My father died about ten years ago," he said. "We weren't very close, so I'm not sure if he ever knew, but I was a teenager when I finally admitted to myself that I was gay. I tried to change at first, but . . . my father never seemed very proud of me, so I spent a lot of time trying to be someone else."

I struggled to keep my eyes on the highway. But when Robert's voice wavered, I couldn't help but glance at him. He looked heartbroken, sitting there with this distant look on his face, as if he were waiting for me to ask why he didn't tell me before the adoption. But I already knew the answer. He was ashamed. I was about to ask if Julie knew, but our minute-long silence answered that question too. She didn't know. It didn't bother me that he was gay. Of course I was surprised. It was the idea of keeping his secret from Julie that worried me. She was my mom now.

But the fact that Robert felt safe enough to confide in me was an incredible gift. Since the day I had met him, he had always supported me. He had guided me through some of the most difficult years of my life. He had been there through the lawsuit and the settlement and my mom abandoning me again. I couldn't help but love him for trusting me enough to keep his secret.

Robert was still looking out the window when he finally spoke again.

"I used to collect comic books when I was a kid," he said. "I'd spend hours daydreaming about being a superhero like Shrinking Violet or Lightning Lad. I knew I'd never develop any special powers, but I was smart enough to be an attorney, and that seemed pretty close to a superhero to me. So when you and Kevin and the other kids decided to sue the hospital, I knew I'd found my chance. I just wanted to save you all. For once I wanted to be a hero to someone."

When I replay that moment in my mind, I don't recall the highway or watching the road. I only remember the sweet smell of pipe tobacco and the image of Robert leaning back against his headrest with tears streaming down his face. Even then I knew those words would forever shape how I saw my new father. A profound gratitude welled up inside me. That afternoon, away from his home and office and family, he wasn't an attorney or an ordained minister. He was just a little kid who wanted someone to be proud of him.

"Hey, Pop," I said.

I waited until he turned to face me. His downcast eyes were red and swollen. I put my hand on his arm to remind both of us that I was still his son.

"You're not just my hero now," I said. "You're my dad too."

12

Jennifer

"K evin was killed in a car accident today," Robert cried over the phone. "You know why they kept Kevin in the hospital? Because he was gay. It could have been me."

Kevin Matthew Mardason died on March 26, 1995. He was twenty-two years old. He had survived nearly three of those years in the hospital and spent months tied to a bed or a wheelchair. Since the end of the lawsuit, Kevin's behavior had grown more erratic. He had started drinking a lot and driving recklessly. Robert had always gone out of his way to help him, but it wasn't until our road trip that I understood why. They had both spent years trying to hide who they truly were.

Robert picked me up later that week and drove us to Restland, a funeral home in Dallas just a few miles from my old apartment and the restaurant where my mom had walked out on our dinner. We parked in front of a small chapel. I was getting out of the car when Robert asked me to wait while he reloaded his pipe and struck a match.

"Ban, when we go inside, there's going to be a girl here you'll probably think is the most beautiful woman you've ever seen." Robert paused and took a few puffs for dramatic emphasis. "Don't talk to her. Her dad's an attorney. And she's an addict."

"You're an attorney," I said.

"You did hear me mention that she's an addict, right?"

I laughed and got out of the car and then walked to the chapel. Robert had already started up a conversation with several kids from the lawsuit, so I stepped inside alone. The foyer was filled with stained-glass windows and people bathed in colorful sunlight. I recognized more than a dozen of them. Most of the others were people whose names I knew, but I'd never met them because we had been held in separate units in the hospital.

Sean, my friend who had been in bed restraints for nearly a year, walked over and gave me a bear hug. Together we walked around the funeral home and reunited with old friends and shared stories about Kevin, about his ridiculous alter egos and how he always managed to laugh at Luther and the doctors. We all loved Kevin for his rebellious happiness.

The funeral lasted less than an hour. I watched Kevin's mother throughout most of it. She looked small and frail, like a doll in a black dress sitting forgotten on a bench somewhere, her lifeless gaze fixed on something far away. Sometimes she'd close her eyes and lower her head and begin to cry. Then someone next to her would put an arm around her and she'd fall silent again.

Soon the minister closed the service and invited everyone to join a ceremony at Kevin's graveside. I shuffled out of the pew and walked down the aisle toward a pair of swinging wooden doors, both of them furnished with rectangular metal hand plates. I don't know why, but I clearly remember setting my palms inside the border of each of them before pushing the doors open.

She was standing in the far corner of the foyer, surveying the room. A long curtain of dark hair fell over her shoulders, and her sleepy feline eyes made her look proud and unapproachable. She wore a black sweater over a blouse and a long black skirt. Her eyes were gilded in meticulous Cleopatra eyeliner. A woman standing next to her looked like her mom.

Wow, Robert was right. She is the most beautiful girl I've ever seen.

A voice spoke from behind me. "Hey, Banning. You make a better door than a window."

I turned to see Sean holding the doors for a group of people I was blocking, so I stepped out of the way and asked him about the girl in the corner.

"That's Jennifer," he said.

"Which one?"

We all knew the two Jennifers from the hospital, improbably named Jennifer Fox and Jennifer Wolfe.

"Fox," Sean said.

I remembered people talking about Jennifer Fox during my first few weeks on the unit. A lot of the kids were upset she had left and that I had taken her place. She was only fourteen when she was admitted, and she spent months in restraints during her two years locked in the hospital. Everyone loved her, especially Kevin.

Sean and I walked to the back of the darkened foyer and waited in line to go outside. Across the room, the doors of the chapel had been propped open, and the sunlight outside painted everyone in shadow. We were nearly to the exit when Jennifer and her mom merged into the line in front of us, and I looked down to see Jennifer's entire figure in shadow against the light in the doorway. The silhouette of her long legs stood behind the veil of her floor-length black skirt. She was wearing heels and rested on one leg while playing with one of her shoes with her bare foot.

A dizzying wave of lust raced through me. I glanced at the people next to me, wondering if they somehow knew what I was thinking. I'd never wanted someone so badly that I could barely breathe.

When the line moved, Sean and I stepped outside and followed the group to the ceremony. I scanned the crowd around Kevin's casket to see Jennifer standing on the far side opposite us. In the cloudy light of late afternoon, she looked even more mysterious than before, her heart-shaped face lowered in prayer.

The minister closed the ceremony and Kevin's casket was lowered into his grave. Then we all paid our last respects to him and his family before gathering in front of the chapel. Robert invited everyone to dinner in Fort Worth. He never mentioned Jennifer on the drive back and I didn't volunteer that I'd seen her.

I spent the hour-long drive composing what I'd say to her, but when we arrived at the restaurant she and her mother were nowhere to be found. Throughout dinner I pushed my food around my plate while Robert and my friends shared stories about Kevin, but all I could think about was Jennifer. I casually asked a few of my friends about her, but her time in the hospital predated most of ours. No one knew her phone number or where she lived, and I knew asking Robert would mean another lecture.

We finished dinner and our group parted ways outside the restaurant. Sean and a couple of other friends from the hospital followed us to Robert and Julie's house, where I'd left my car. I wanted to be alone, so I wandered back to the study and deflated into Robert's office chair while I tried to think of some way to see Jennifer again, but it seemed pointless. The only person who knew her was Robert, and he wasn't about to give me her phone number.

I was about to get up and join everyone in the living room when I noticed a familiar green binder lying under a pile of books. I'd fetched it for Robert dozens of times. Printed inside were the phone numbers and addresses of everyone who had been a part of the lawsuit, including Jennifer.

It was after midnight when I finally got the courage to call Jennifer. Tundra lay asleep on the bed and I sat next to her and dialed the number I'd stolen from Robert's study. The line rang twice and then stopped. I could hear voices on a television in the background.

"Who is this?" Jennifer asked.

"I can't tell you."

I sound like a fucking stalker.

"Then I'm going to hang up," she said.

"Wait, I've wanted to talk to you for hours and now I don't know what to say." I took a breath and closed my eyes. "You're the most beautiful woman I've ever seen. All I can do is think of you. I couldn't even eat dinner tonight. I didn't even want to. I just wanted to see you again."

"If you don't tell me who this is, I'm going to hang up."

"No, you won't," I said. "Then you'll lay in bed all night, wondering."

She asked if I'd seen her that day. I thought about lying for a moment, but it seemed childish, so I said yes.

"Well, there's only a few places I could have seen you," she said. "I flew back home today to go to my friend's funeral. Then I went to dinner with my mom." She paused as if she were replaying the day in her mind. "Is this the guy from the plane?"

I glared at the phone. "You gave some random guy on a plane your number?"

"He was cute, but he was too old for me," she said, ignoring my comment. "He asked me out, but I told him I'm dating someone."

I cringed. "Are you dating someone?"

"No, I broke up with my boyfriend a couple of months ago."

"Why did you break up with him?" I asked.

"Because he's a fucking asshole."

I looked at Tundra and pointed at myself. "I'm not an asshole. I'm super sweet."

"Just tell me who this is," she said. "I think I know who you are, and . . ."

"And what?"

"I'm not telling you. You called me."

"If you can guess who I am, then I'll tell you if you're right," I said.

She asked for a hint and I told her my name started with a *B*. The phone went quiet.

"But Banning," she said. "I'm damaged merchandise."

I lay back on my bed and stared at the ceiling. "We were both in the hospital. If you're damaged merchandise, then I am too."

There was a long moment of silence. I began to wonder if I had said the wrong thing. I was about to apologize when Jennifer began recounting the nightmares and panic attacks that had plagued her since she left the hospital. There was a quiet secret in her voice, as if she hadn't shared those memories in a long time. I sat on the floor next to my bed and listened to her tell stories about people and things like we had lived the same life. She remembered Kevin and Sonia and the way staff would look through the windows when they were about to rush someone. She remembered Luther's black shoes and the blue plastic covers on our charts.

Then she described the first time she was held down by a group of orderlies and put in restraints when she was fourteen years old. I told her about the first time I went outside, when I stood in my socks in the sunlight and listened to the birds and the highway. We spent hours laughing and crying and sharing stories. When she finally confessed to getting into heroin and prescription drugs to deal with her memories of the hospital and being in restraints, all I could think to say was "It's okay." Because even though her admission scared me, through my wounded twenty-three-year-old eyes, everything about Jennifer was perfect.

"You were so cute today," she said. "You looked like a professor in your brown wool suit. I kept hoping you'd notice me and smile."

"I was staring at you the whole time. I remember watching you walk out of the chapel. God, you were so beautiful."

She was quiet for a moment. "Do you still think I'm beautiful?"

We talked until six in the morning, when the sky was growing light. Before going to sleep, I finally asked what I had wanted to ask her all day. "Would you like to have dinner tomorrow?"

"It is tomorrow," she said. "And yes. Tonight."

We met that afternoon at Whole Foods on Greenville Avenue. It was April Fools' Day. I arrived ten minutes early and walked up and down every aisle while I strangled a dozen roses in one hand. Twenty minutes passed. Then thirty.

There's no way she's going to show up. A girl like her would never go out with me. It's probably some April Fools' joke.

I fished my keys out of my pocket and started walking to my car.

"I'm so sorry. It took me forever to get ready."

I turned to see Jennifer standing about ten feet away. Her almond-shaped hazel eyes narrowed with a smile. She wore a pair of heels and a short dress decorated with small blue flowers. A long curtain of charcoal brown hair fell over her shoulders.

"I couldn't decide what to wear," she said, looking down at herself.

She waited for me to say something, but I just stood there and stared at her. A shy smile curled her lips when she noticed the cellophane-wrapped bouquet in my hand.

"Roses," she said.

I glanced at the flowers. "Oh yeah, these are for you."

She stepped toward me and draped her arms around my neck and gave me a hug. I closed my eyes and held her as she leaned into me.

"I'm glad you called," she whispered.

We spent half an hour wandering the store. We read get-well cards to each other and argued about the best combinations of bulk candy. She laced her fingers through mine when I told her that she smelled nice, then pinched my arm when I said I liked dogs more than cats. She never asked where I worked or why I didn't have a job. She didn't seem to care that I sometimes looked away when I needed to articulate something important. My mind never badgered me with thoughts or feelings I needed to hide. If there were other people in the store, I didn't notice them. Jennifer was all that I could see.

We were standing in the checkout line when she began digging through her purse.

"I got this for you," she said, "to remember our first date."

It was a Pez dispenser. I looked at the character through the clear plastic package.

"Oh, hey, it's Goofy," I said.

Jennifer's eyes frosted over. "That is *not* Goofy. It's Pluto. Everyone confuses them. Just remember that Pluto never talks. He's a dog. Nobody likes Goofy. He's fucking creepy."

We left the store to walk down the street to a small Italian restaurant. She asked if I wanted a glass of wine before remembering the straight-edge tattoo on my hand. I told her I didn't care about being sober anymore. "I got that when I was seventeen," I said. "I needed something to be proud of. That was all I had." She smiled and wrapped her arm around mine. I knew she struggled with addiction, and I wanted her to know that I didn't judge her for it. Besides, I wasn't about to refuse to drink if it meant losing her.

The hostess seated us at a candlelit table covered in white linen. A grin flashed across Jennifer's face when I asked our waiter for another glass of whatever wine she had ordered.

"So you've never done any drugs?" she asked. "Smoked weed? Nothing?"

I shook my head. "I was always too busy skating or playing drums."

She stared at the tablecloth in silence. The candlelight and her Cleopatra eyeliner made her look like a mysterious fortune teller.

"I'm not sure you know what you're getting into," she said.

"The hospital fucked up all of us. We all deal with it in our own way. If anyone understands, it's me."

It was long after dark when we left the restaurant. We held hands and wandered past shops filled with smoking incense and bars crowded with people. Moths fluttered in wild circles around the fluorescent street-lights above us. We were walking across the parking lot toward our cars when I stopped to look at her. I held her hand and smiled, but I didn't say anything. I wanted to remember the moment.

"I wish tonight didn't have to end," I said.

She smiled and squeezed my hand. "I live just down the street."

I followed Jennifer's car to her house two blocks away. The building's old hardwood floors creaked when we stepped inside. She had just closed the door behind us and turned on the hallway light when a black cat slunk into the entryway to greet her. It froze and then glared at me.

"Come here, Nunu. Banning's sweet," Jennifer said. "Even though he doesn't like cats."

She picked him up and cradled his long, sleek body before holding his face and kissing him. The cat cringed and hopped to the floor. Then he flicked his tail and walked away.

"Let me grab a couple of glasses of wine," she said. "Make yourself at home."

I stepped into a small living room. Dresses and skirts and shoes lay scattered all over the room. An aluminum can sat upside down on the coffee table next to a lighter and an ashtray. Its scorched bottom had been punctured with a small hole.

I wonder what that's for. Probably smoking weed.

"Turn on the TV," Jennifer said from the kitchen. "We can curl up on the sofa and watch something."

I was thumbing through the channels when she returned, so I settled for MTV. She placed two glasses of wine on the coffee table and then kicked off her heels and sat down. The inches of space between us made me lightheaded and dizzy. She turned to look at me. The television painted her face in ever-changing colors.

"What?" I asked.

She didn't answer. She just smiled and kept her eyes fixed on mine. For minutes one of us would laugh and the other would follow, until our laughter settled into a long gaze filled with all the things we weren't willing to share. A shy grin crept across her lips. She closed her eyes and looked away as something rattled across her teeth.

"What was that?"

She stuck out her tongue to reveal a silver piercing.

I winced. "Damn, I bet that hurt."

"Getting it's not that bad," she said. "It's the next day or two that's painful. I had to eat soup and ice cream. My tongue was really swollen."

We grew quiet again and stared at each other. Finally my wild urge to touch Jennifer overwhelmed the little self-control I had left. My heart began to race as I skimmed my fingers across her knees. She leaned toward me and looked from one of my eyes to the other.

"Can I kiss you?" she asked.

I was about to answer when she wrapped her arms around my neck and pushed me back against the sofa. Then, with her mouth barely open, she grazed the tip of her tongue across my closed lips.

"There's no way I'm letting you go home tonight," she said.

13.

Alligator Food

I cracked my eyes to see a thin white curtain and the silhouette of a mockingbird singing in a tree outside the window. Jennifer lay curled up in front of me, her naked skin smooth and warm.

"Can we stay in bed all day?" she whispered.

That morning was the first of nearly three weeks of mornings that Jennifer and I spent together. The few nights we slept apart, we stayed on the phone until we fell asleep. I'd wake up in the middle of the night or the morning and search through my sheets to find the phone so I could listen to the slow, soft rhythm of her breath.

Neither of us had a job or any obligations after the lawsuit. We spent days wandering through museums and watching movies and making love, like two teenagers who had survived the end of the world. Everything about Jennifer fascinated me. Whenever we stopped at Baskin-Robbins, she'd order a kid's cup of frosting instead of ice cream. Sometimes I'd wake up in the middle of the night to find her whispering Mazzy Star or

Billie Holiday songs in my ear. During one of our first visits to the museum, she spent half an hour contemplating a painting by Mondrian before walking away in silence.

"What do you like about it?" I asked.

She stopped and turned to gaze at the painting's faded gray and brown geometry. She looked like a rainy Sunday morning, quiet and still in her long black dress. For a moment, it seemed like she might say something. Then, without a word, she shrugged and smiled and walked away.

All the worst moments of my life were worth the happiness of those days.

Robert's initial warning about Jennifer evolved into cautious optimism. The two of them had grown close during the lawsuit, and Robert explained that his initial warning about her being an addict wasn't just for my sake; it was for Jennifer's sake as well.

"You're intense, Ban. You know what you want," Robert said, rolling some dice during one of our games of D&D. "Jennifer's twenty-three. She's working through a lot of stuff right now. If you want things to work out, you're going to need to be patient."

I slumped over the table and onto my books. "I know. I'm just crazy about her. I don't know what to do."

"She's crazy about you too. I don't think she'd mind my telling you."

"You still talk to her?" I asked.

"Of course, but I'm not going to betray her trust, or yours. You both can come to me about anything. I won't discuss it with anyone else, including either of you." He looked up from his book. "Remember, Jennifer's an addict. I'm not saying that in judgment. It's simply a fact. She knows it and I know it. And it's important that you know it too."

I leaned back in my chair but didn't say anything.

"Have you talked to her about it?" he asked.

"She said she still smokes heroin sometimes."

"It sounds like you both need to have a longer talk."

"What am I supposed to do," I asked, "just sit down and talk to her about drug abuse?"

"Ban, if you two are as serious about one another as you both say, this won't be your last difficult talk about something important." Robert scanned his notes before rolling another handful of dice. "No matter how successful she is in fighting her demons, she's always going to struggle with what happened in the hospital. You can't ignore that."

It was the middle of April when Jennifer invited me to meet her parents. They lived in a small town called McKinney, a rural suburb more than an hour away. She had asked them if I could stay the night, so they agreed to put me up in the guest bedroom for the weekend.

The next day we parked in front of a large two-story house in a private community. Tall, lush trees shaded the grass of a fairway and golf course behind the homes across the street. The neighborhood looked like a movie set, with streets lined with perfect houses and meticulous lawns. A bright red convertible parked in a driveway jarred loose a memory of my dad waxing a similar car and waving to me from a life that wasn't mine anymore. But when Jennifer stopped at the door and turned around to reach for my hand, I remembered that being with her was all that mattered to me now.

Jennifer's dad was tall and thin, and he smiled when he shook my hand. I recognized her mom from the funeral. She had dark hair and green eyes, and her New Jersey accent made me wonder whether she was friendly or brutally honest or both. She introduced herself as Cecilia before giving me a hug.

I followed Jennifer upstairs and left my bag in the guest room where I'd be staying. A shared bathroom separated our rooms. Her four-poster bed was a three-second walk from where I'd be sleeping. I could see it from my pillow.

"My parents never come upstairs," she said with a smile.

We left the house and wandered barefoot around the golf course, watching the sky change color with the sunset. Sometimes I'd stop and watch Jennifer walk ahead, and I'd record the moment in my mind like I had so many others. She seemed so mysterious, with her dark hair and hazel eyes and closely held secrets. Even her drug abuse was alluring. Its naked, obvious destruction looked almost like courage compared with my always wanting to be normal again. I had spent years trying to understand the hell that Jennifer and I had survived. She had simply torched the wreckage and walked away.

It was dusk by the time we stopped on one of the greens. The grass was wet and the back of my jeans grew damp as I sat and stared at the dark blue sky. Jennifer pushed my knees apart with one of her bare feet before sitting down and reclining against my chest. She set her shoes next to us.

The golf course was surrounded by houses hidden behind a fence. The green canopy of an oak tree hovered over the backyard of one of them. Its leaves stirred in the breeze as Jennifer leaned back against me and pulled my arms around her. I ran my lips over the back of her neck.

"Alligator food," she said.

"Alligator food?"

"Watch me say it," she said, turning around to face me. She mouthed the words again and it looked like she had said, "I love you."

I pushed her backward and she stretched out underneath me with her eyes fixed on mine. Beads of dew dotted the grass around us. She wrapped her legs around my waist.

"We could make love right here," she whispered. "In the dark."

No one had ever made me feel as hungry for someone as Jennifer. It didn't matter where we were or what we were doing; she only needed to smile or narrow her eyes and I was her plaything. But I never understood the joy of making someone feel good until I met her. We would lock eyes while we made love and she would smile and laugh or claw my arms and back. The ferocity of her pleasure was unlike anything I'd ever experienced. I never knew I could make someone so happy.

Jennifer lay in the grass between my hands and knees, watching me as I planted a trail of kisses down her body until I was lying between her legs. I slid my hands underneath her skirt to find her naked from the waist down. She closed her eyes and drew a breath as the tip of my tongue grazed the base of her small, trimmed patch of hair. The smooth skin below it was warm and wet and sweet. She arched her back and pushed herself against my lips.

My elbows sank into the wet grass as she writhed against my mouth. I held still and let her find her own rhythm. Her hands searched for mine. Then she wove our fingers together before grinding the soft pearl of her clitoris against my tongue and lips. With her back arched and arms locked, she cried out while her body seized in long waves of tension and release. I had pressed my mouth against her, hoping to prolong her orgasm, when she began to cry.

It wasn't the first time Jennifer had cried during an orgasm, but there was something different about this time. Instead of collapsing in relief or quietly rolling onto her side, she lay in the grass for nearly ten minutes while she trembled and wept. The entire neighborhood around us was still, as if the world had fallen silent out of respect for whatever she was experiencing. I tried kissing her legs and stomach, but even the slightest sensation made her convulse and grasp for my hands. I sat in the grass next to her, trying to imagine what she was feeling while her chest rose and fell ever more slowly. I began to wonder if I had done something wrong.

She opened her eyes and stared at the sky. The corners of her lips curled into a delicate smile when she finally looked at me.

"You okay?" I asked.

She lowered her chin in a gentle nod. Her smile widened.

I got to my feet and offered her my hand. Instead of taking it, she lay there and stared at me standing between her and the night sky. She didn't say anything. She just watched me with her head rolled to the side and a smile in her eyes like a child contemplating the stars. I wanted to ask her what she was thinking, but I knew she wouldn't tell me, and I didn't want to ruin the moment.

Eventually she took my hand and I pulled her to her feet. Without a word, she straightened her dress and then grabbed her shoes and began walking back toward her parents' house. I was about to ask her what had happened when she stopped and squeezed my hand. She could have put her finger to my lips, but she simply smiled and stared at me, as if to let me know that sometimes it was better to be silent when the world was silent too.

———

The house was quiet when I woke the next morning. Jennifer and I had fallen asleep together, so I snuck back into the guest room before sunrise. A couple of hours later I crawled out of bed and wandered downstairs. The living room was warm and bright and the sliding glass door was open, and a song playing on a radio drifted in from outside. I squinted my eyes to see Jennifer sitting on the patio with her legs in the swimming pool. She turned to the side and set her foot next to a bottle of baby oil and a razor.

"Are you shaving your legs in the pool?" I asked through the screen.

She turned and looked at me. "Yeah. Are you spying on your girlfriend?"

There was an easiness in her words that made my heart race. I knew Jennifer cared for me, but sometimes her solitude left me feeling small and unimportant. Robert had warned me about her drug abuse. Jennifer and I had even talked about it. But everything I had imagined about falling in love with an addict never happened. There were no empty medicine bottles or overdoses or burned spoons. There were only moments of silence hiding something I couldn't quite understand.

I stepped onto the patio and into the sunlight. The warm concrete felt nice under my feet, so I hiked up my pajamas and sat next to Jennifer before lowering my legs into the cold water.

"Doesn't shaving in the pool make a mess?" I asked.

"I don't know," she said. "Nobody uses it. My dad keeps it clean."

When I asked if her parents were home, she said they had gone to church. I'd sat back on my elbows and was watching her shave when another question fluttered out of the back of my mind.

"What's heroin feel like?"

I had never thought about drugs until I met Jennifer. Other than the occasional whiff of weed at a show, I had no experience with them. The only time I'd ever listened to anyone talk about drug abuse was in the halfway house, and even then it was in retrospect. I'd watched those friends struggle with addiction every day. And I could relate to that, indirectly, because drugs weren't the real problem; it was trauma or abuse that made them appealing. But that morning, while I sat next to Jennifer with my question still hanging in the air, whatever reaction I expected—anger, silence, a raised eyebrow—never arrived. She just shook her razor in the pool and stared at the water.

"Heroin's hard to explain," she said. "It's like getting in a warm bath and staying underwater. Everything's soft and quiet." A smile crept across her lips, as if she were recalling an old friend. "It's really nice."

"Did you do it before the hospital?" I asked.

She shook her head. "I kept having nightmares after I left, about getting rushed and being in restraints. That's when I first started having panic attacks. I'd only been out of the hospital for a month or two when I tried it for the first time."

"How long were you in restraints?"

She shrugged. "A few weeks. I don't know."

We fell quiet and she wiped her legs with a towel. She kept her eyes fixed on her hands. I felt terrible for mentioning the hospital on such a beautiful morning.

"My therapist finally put me on Xanax," she said. "I still take it sometimes, but it keeps me from having orgasms, so I started taking Rohypnol instead."

I'd never heard of Rohypnol. Jennifer had to spell it for me. For some reason that made it seem more dangerous than heroin, though I don't know why. I didn't want to look concerned, so I stared at my feet. Jennifer fell quiet again and hugged her knees to her chest, her eyes still looking away.

"A couple of years after I got out of the hospital, I went to a party with a friend," she said. "We shot up in one of the bedrooms. The next thing I remember, he was raping me."

She looked at me. I didn't know what to say. I felt like the wind had been kicked out of me. I could feel my heartbeat in my face.

"I just laid there," she said, "staring at the wall. I didn't even try to push him off me. It's like I was just lying there watching it happen." She rested her forehead on her knees and began to cry. "I still feel like it's my fault."

I scooted closer and reached out to touch her.

"Don't," she said, leaning away.

I searched for something to say, but the words in my mind sounded meaningless and stupid. I felt helpless. She glanced at me from behind her knees while I sat there wondering what to do. Then she gave up and hid her face and began to cry again.

"I don't know what to say," I told her, fighting my urge to touch her. "I just wish I could help."

She hugged her knees and wept, her dark hair trailing down her oily legs, like long brushstrokes of ink on smooth paper.

"Just listening and not leaving's good," she said.

"I'll never leave you, no matter what happens. Remember the first time I called you? When you said you were damaged merchandise? I loved it when you said that. I know what it's like to feel broken, but you're perfect to me. I wouldn't change anything about you."

Jennifer smiled and then wiped her eyes. "But I'm still using," she said.

"I don't care."

"You should. Even if I stop, I'll just fuck up and do it again. I've done that for years. I've probably stopped twenty times."

"Then we can go to meetings together or something," I said. "All my friends in the halfway house went to NA and AA. They loved it."

Nothing she could say would change my mind. I wasn't going to stop falling in love with my best friend because she was an addict. I'd help her, the same way Robert had helped me.

I stood and offered her my hand. She grabbed my wrist and then got to her feet.

"My parents won't be home for a while," she said. "Let's go take a shower."

An hour later we were lying in bed, laughing and talking as if the morning hadn't happened and we had just woken up. She draped one of her smooth legs over mine and I looked down the length of our bodies to see her wearing a pair of white ruffled socks.

"You always wear socks," I said. "How can your feet be cold?"

"They're cozy. I just like wearing them." She leaned over me and grazed her fingers across my wrist. "You have such beautiful arms," she said. "Mine are all fucked up and ugly now." She lifted one of them and held it close to my face. A faint trail of scars traced her veins.

She's testing me.

I took her hand and ran my lips from the inside of her wrist to her elbow. She combed her fingers through my hair while I kissed her arm.

"There," I said. "They're all gone now. See?"

Her eyes smiled. She pointed at a freckle. "You missed one."

The house where Jennifer lived with her cat and perpetually absent roommate stood in the heart of Dallas, a city filled with memories of the worst years of my life. So when April came to an end and Jennifer began going home for days at a time, I was reluctant to join her. It wasn't until she insisted on my coming to stay for the weekend that I finally caught a glimpse of her other life.

Jennifer loved people and adored her friends. A few of them were women, but most turned out to be flamboyant gay men who reminded me of Kevin.

"Girls are catty and mean," she once told me. "Everything's a fucking competition with them. Guys are simple. What you see is what you get."

I spent most of our evenings in Dallas driving Jennifer from one bar to the next, where she would wiggle into the middle of a booth and sit surrounded by her friends, like some gothic princess holding court. She would giggle and gossip and comfort her friends. She would shout over them and then hug and kiss them. Then we would bid her audience farewell and walk to the car while she talked about how nice it was to see everyone again. I loved seeing Jennifer happy, and I liked meeting her friends, but socializing was exhausting for me. My mind insisted on decoding every word and action. Jennifer thrived around people, until she had had enough. Then, instead of gesturing toward the next bar, she would recline the passenger seat and point at the windshield and tell me to take her home or back to my apartment so we could be alone.

Jennifer had another group of friends. All of them called her Jenna.

Sometimes they would stop by her house and smoke some weed and I'd leave the room and read a book until they went home. Other times I'd call late at night and they would hand the phone to Jennifer and she would sneak off to her room and say how much she missed me. Sometimes she fell asleep. Other nights someone might come to check on her and she would cover the phone and say something to them before telling me she needed to go. Then she would call back in the middle of the night and curl up in bed and whisper to me while she drifted off to sleep.

I never told Jennifer how much those nights hurt me, how I would lie there in the dark and stare at the ceiling while my heart slowly broke. I wanted her to spend time with me, not people who only stopped by when they wanted to drink or smoke some weed. I couldn't stand those people. They were shadows to me, figments of my fear and insecurity. For hours my mind would chase itself, trying to predict how Jennifer might leave me someday, until I grew so anxious the room began to spin. I suppose I should have told her that I was afraid of losing her. But after being abandoned by my mom and dad, I didn't want to do anything that would make her leave me. I had lost enough in my life. Being honest wasn't worth losing her too.

By the end of May we had made an appointment to get tested for HIV. Robert had hassled me about it since my first date with Jennifer nearly two months before. But every time I tried bringing it up to her, the words lodged in my throat like a clump of rocks.

I don't care if I get HIV, I decided. *I'd rather have a disease with Jennifer than live my life without her.*

Eventually she mentioned the idea of getting tested on her own, so I volunteered to go with her. I felt like a coward. It took a week to get the results. Every day I woke up with a knot in my stomach, wondering what I'd say if we tested positive.

Did you share a needle? Are you still using? Are you going to leave me?

But when the results came back negative, those questions didn't matter anymore, so I forgot about them.

We went to dinner to celebrate at a small Italian restaurant in a basement in Fort Worth. Jennifer wore a long black dress that almost touched the floor. The dining room had a grand piano, a candle on every table, and doors on the booths for privacy. She held my hand while we looked at the menu, and I could feel the lacy tops of her stockings through her skirt. When we left, the few people still in the restaurant turned to watch her sail toward the exit.

It was late that night when she crawled out of bed, naked except for her beloved socks. She turned on the faucet before using the bathroom. "The sound helps me pee," she said. I watched her walk back to bed in the glow of the streetlight outside my bedroom window. She curled up next to me.

"Do you think we're codependent?" she asked.

We laughed. The term had been used so often in the hospital that it became a joke. None of us were ever put in restraints for being codependent. Sometimes patients projected their feelings. Others were in denial. But most of us, at one time or another, had been told we were codependent. Yet no one ever explained what caused it or how to treat it.

I pulled the sheets over us. "I don't know. Aren't we supposed to need other people?"

She shrugged.

"Didn't they explain it to you?" I asked.

"They put me in restraints right after my parents signed me in to the hospital," she said. "I didn't really give a fuck about therapy after that."

Jennifer was in seventh grade when her parents put her in the hospital. She had wanted a dress for a dance, so they took her to the mall to go shopping.

"I walked out of the dressing room and my mom freaked out," Jennifer told me. "She said I looked like a bag lady. We got into a screaming match in the middle of the store, so I went home and locked myself in my room and said I was going to slit my wrists." She shook her head and laughed. "I was such a drama queen. Mom called some doctor and he had me signed in to the hospital the next day. I'd never even seen him before. Mom and Dad didn't know him either. They were just scared."

Jennifer trailed off into silence before asking why my parents signed me in to the hospital. I recounted the entire story. Giving away my skateboard. My school counselor in her car. Watching Sam in the nurses' station. Then I told her about going on passes and the bowling alley and getting so angry that sometimes I imagined I'd turn into Sonia, and that all the pain and rage I had witnessed in the hospital had somehow infected me.

"But didn't you get mad before the hospital?" Jennifer asked.

"Yeah, but it was different back then. I still remember when anger felt normal, like something I could hold in my hands and control, like a Rubik's Cube." I twisted my hands as if I were manipulating the little puzzle. "But after the hospital it didn't feel like anger anymore. It felt dangerous, like it's bigger and stronger than me now."

"I can get really mad sometimes," she said. "I'll scream and yell, but that's not what I'm really feeling. Usually I'm just sad. Sometimes I feel like the doctors removed something inside of me." She rolled onto her back and laid her hand on her stomach. "Like a happinessectomy."

She lay there for a moment and stared at the ceiling. Then she got out of bed and walked across the room and flicked on the lights. Everything went white. I shut my eyes.

"You want to know why I always wear socks?" she said, sitting down next to me.

I sat up and leaned back against the cold wooden headboard of my sleigh bed. She set one of her feet on top of the covers and spread her toes to reveal a small cluster of dark dots.

"Those are from shooting up," she said.

It was another test. I'd passed dozens of her tests. I was tired of them. I was tired of the silence and doubt and worry. Sometimes I wanted to be tired of her. But my heart had picked Jennifer and left me to find my way out of her maze.

I ran a finger over the dots between her toes. "Doesn't it hurt to shoot up there?" I asked.

"Of course it hurts, dummy," she said.

I didn't know what else to say. I felt small and childish compared with Jennifer, especially when I tried to understand her drug abuse. It terrified me. Maybe because she loved it. Maybe because I wanted to destroy myself too. But whatever the reason, whenever she forced me to stare into that dark place inside her, I wanted to run away, until I remembered that she didn't do heroin because wanted to. She did it because of the hospital.

I walked to the light switch and flicked it down and then stood there in the darkness. Jennifer began crying.

"You're going to leave me someday," she said. "I know you will."

I walked back to the bed and sat down.

"I'll never leave you," I said. "I love you."

She rolled over and faced the wall. "No, you don't. You love what you think I am."

I set my hand on her back and closed my eyes. I imagined drawing her pain and suffering through my hand and into me, where I could turn it into something beautiful.

She spoke after a long time. "Do you think we'll ever not be fucked up?"

I laughed. "No."

"But what if we're always like this?" she said, rolling over to face me.

"Then we'll be fucked up together. It's better than being normal without you."

The next morning Jennifer went home. We didn't see each other for nearly two weeks. Instead, we talked on the phone every night and she sent me lipstick-kissed notes in the mail. I drove to her house every few days and left a dozen roses on her doorstep, but I never rang the doorbell. We fell asleep on the phone while we watched movies together. Robert said she called him, but he never offered anything more than to say she was working through a difficult time and that she loved me.

"Give her a couple of weeks," he said. "She just needs some space. If you push, you'll only drive her away."

I had never been in love before I met Jennifer, let alone with someone who had shared so much with me. Until I'd met her, the hospital seemed like a curse, but it bound us together. It helped us understand things about ourselves we had never understood before, like how we both loved being touched because we had lived without it for so long. But I was afraid of how deeply I loved her. When we were apart, I felt like I'd been turned inside out. My bones ached. My heart raced. I didn't want to sleep or eat. It took all my effort not to pick up the phone and call her. Our time apart scared me. Her addiction felt like an old lover who was constantly asking her to leave me. I was jealous and afraid of it. But I knew Robert was right; I knew I had to let Jennifer go and wait for her to come back to me when she was ready.

I returned to my computer to distract myself. I was lost in a game one afternoon when Jennifer called and asked if I had ever seen *When Harry Met Sally*. I said I hadn't, so she told me to turn on my TV and set it to whatever channel she was watching. For two hours I sat on the floor with Tundra while Jennifer narrated the entire movie, even when I asked her to stop. She laughed until she couldn't speak when Meg Ryan faked her orgasm, and she cried at the end when Billy Crystal declared his love for her. Jennifer repeated the line in unison with him.

"I came here tonight because when you realize you want to spend the rest of your life with somebody, you want the rest of your life to start as soon as possible."

"That's how I feel about you," she said. "I want to be with you forever. I don't want to lose you."

"You're not going to lose me."

"I'm scared though," she said.

"Of what?"

"I don't know. I'm just scared, like something's going to go wrong."

"Well, if something does go wrong," I said, "at least we'll always have each other."

14.

A Girl in a Silent Film

It was June. Spring was nearly over and the weather had grown warm and humid. I gave Jennifer a key to my apartment and sometimes I'd wake up to her crawling into bed next to me with her skin warm and salty from the sunlight. Our two week "break," as she called it, had come to an end with the credits of *When Harry Met Sally*, followed by a long talk about my being too intense and a promise that she would take her drug abuse seriously.

"You love me too much," she told me once. "It's scary. I need for things to be fun and easy sometimes."

I couldn't understand why Jennifer didn't want love and intensity all the time, but I knew I'd lose her if I didn't give her space. I quit calling every night. I stopped asking what she had done on our days apart. Then, when I found out one of my favorite bands was playing a show in Fort Worth, I invited her to come with me.

It'll be a chance to do something fun and easy, I thought.

It was warm and windy that weekend. Jennifer stayed over the night before the show, and the next day we drove through downtown Fort Worth with the windows down. She held my hand while we talked and laughed over the sound of the wind. We parked in a narrow alley and walked to dinner with her hair drifting behind her like a long dark cloak. Her smile was as bright as the stars. Everything seemed perfect.

The opening band had just finished their set when we strolled past two friends who recalled my years playing for Hagfish. They wondered what had become of me. "You just vanished," one of the guys said. I didn't like being associated with the band and my years in Dallas, so I told them I'd moved to Fort Worth to be near my family. It wasn't a lie.

"I heard you sued a hospital or something," said the other guy.

Jennifer squeezed my hand and then walked to a nearby staircase and sat down. She cast an icy gaze at my friends before glancing at me. I could almost read her mind.

This is our night. Let's just have fun.

The quieter of the two guys craned his neck and searched the crowd. "Hey, Chad's here," he said. He tugged his friend by the shirt and winced in apology as they walked away. When I turned to look at Jennifer, I could tell we were thinking the same thing, as if she had scribbled the words in repetition on a foggy window.

The hospital. The hospital. The hospital.

Sometimes it seemed like the hospital would follow us forever.

I sat next to Jennifer and picked at my shoelaces while the next band took the stage. Everyone inside the venue erupted in applause, but Jennifer and I were miles away. She stood and dusted off her skirt.

"My stomach's bugging me again," she said. "Is there another bathroom around here? The one inside's disgusting."

"There's another around the corner, I think. Do you want me to go with you?"

She shook her head and gave me a kiss and said she would be right back. I walked to the side of the venue and stood in the doorway to watch the band. They were twenty minutes into their set when I circled the building to look for Jennifer. By the time I returned, someone had taken my place, so I scanned the crowd over their shoulder and saw her sitting on a staircase next to the stage. She was leaning against the wall, smiling as she slowly waved to me.

I smiled and waved back, but she didn't seem to notice. She kept weaving her hand through the air, her eyes distant and empty, like a girl in a silent film waving from another time.

She shot up.

I walked through the crowd while Jennifer's eyes trailed behind me, staring at where I'd been moments before. She seemed to be somewhere else, submerged in her bathtub of warm water where everything was safe.

"Are you okay?" I asked.

Her eyes finished tracing the path I'd taken as her memory followed a breadcrumb trail of moments past. She opened her mouth to speak. Her words were dull and disconnected. She could barely open her eyes.

"I love you so much," she said.

"What happened?" The question sounded stupid, but I didn't know what else to say.

A meaningless smile crept across her lips.

"Nothing," she murmured. "Everything's fine."

I helped her to her feet and she leaned on my arm as we stumbled through the crowd. She looked half asleep, shuffling forward with her chin down and her eyes closed and her hair hanging in her face, her body limp. People stepped out of our way to watch her pass.

"Jesus, she's really fucked up," someone said.

The ten-minute walk to the car took half an hour. I was buckling Jennifer into the passenger seat when a couple strolled by and stopped to watch me. I felt like I was kidnapping her.

"Where are we?" Jennifer asked. "Where are we going?"

I told her we were going home, but she kept nodding off and waking up and asking the same question over and over. When we pulled up in front of my apartment, I helped her out of the car before guiding her upstairs. Tundra sat in the bedroom doorway, watching us. Jennifer spent five minutes trying to unzip the back of her dress. Then she gave up and collapsed face down on the bed like she had been shot in the back.

"Are you okay?" I asked. "You didn't overdose, did you?"

She rolled over and looked at me and smiled.

"No, dummy," she said. Her eyelids trembled and she closed her eyes. "Stop talking and lie down."

I helped her out of her clothes and then tucked her into bed. I stayed up for hours, stroking her hair and checking on her. Her breathing seemed normal. I almost called Robert, but Jennifer finally got up in the middle of the night and turned on the faucet to pee. "Thanks for being sweet to me," she said. Then she gave me a kiss and fell back to sleep. When we woke up the next morning, she told me what had happened.

"I shot up in the bathroom," she said. "It was stupid. I'm sorry."

She wasn't testing me this time. She wasn't watching my reaction or waiting for me to say something. She just lay curled up under the sheets, speaking to me as if she were behind a confessional curtain.

"I was okay until we ran into that guy who mentioned the hospital," she said. "I started having a panic attack in the bathroom. I couldn't breathe." She rolled over and reached for her purse on the floor, even though it was ten feet away. "Can you grab my bag for me, please? My stomach's killing me."

"What do you need?" I asked.

She glared at me over her shoulder. "A fucking Imodium."

I crawled over her and fetched her purse. She rummaged through it before retrieving a candy tin filled with an assortment of what clearly was not candy. She tossed a pill in her mouth and then reached for the glass I had set on the nightstand and took a sip of water.

"I'm sorry," she said. "I don't know why I shot up. It was stupid."

I answered without thinking. "It's okay."

She turned and looked at me, still holding the glass.

"You don't get it, do you?" she said. "I shot up last night and you're sitting here telling me it's okay. Don't be so fucking stupid. It's not okay. *I'm* not okay." Jennifer set down the glass and held up her arm and pointed at her trail of scars. "Do you have these?" She grabbed my arm and glanced at it and then shoved it back at me. "No. You don't, because you're mister fucking straight edge."

She pushed herself out of bed and began gathering her clothes from the floor.

"Jennifer, stop," I said. "Please don't leave."

"What are you going to tell me? The same fucking bullshit? That you love me? That love can fix this? Fix *me*? I love you, Banning, but you can't fix me. I'm fucking broken."

She stepped into her dress and pulled it up and left the back unfastened and open, holding it over one shoulder as she collected her things before storming downstairs.

I managed to pull on a pair of boxers and a shirt. I made it to the front door by the time she had found her keys.

"Please don't leave," I said, tearing up. "I don't want to live without you."

She stepped toward me and then stopped a few feet away. If any love or anger remained inside her, it was impossible to see it in her empty gaze.

"I love you, Banning. I've never loved anyone like I love you. That's why I'm leaving."

She opened the door and her shadow passed through a long wedge of sunlight. Then she was gone.

That night I drove to Jennifer's house and left a dozen roses on her doorstep. I called the next morning and left a message on her machine, begging her to talk to me. Two days and another dozen roses later, she finally called in the middle of the night. I was barely awake when she asked to come see me. She sounded sorry, even though she never said the word.

"I miss you," she whispered. "I miss Tundra too."

We spent the rest of the week together, going to the botanical garden and walking under the magnolia trees and sharing our dreams instead of arguing with each other.

"I want to get married someday," I said, "but I'm scared. I don't even know what it's like to have a family. I was a little boy when I had parents. Then they left me at the airport. Every time you storm out on me, I feel like I'm there again. You can't keep doing that."

Jennifer hooked her pinky around mine.

"I want to marry you someday too," she said. "And yeah, it's scary. You're intense. You know exactly what you want. And you're always saying how much you love me, like it's going to make everything better, but it just makes me want to run away."

As those warm weeks of July passed, we realized that neither of us had ever built a real relationship. I craved love and affirmation. Jennifer wanted freedom. She stormed out of arguments because she hated feeling suffocated. I always stopped at the door and threatened to walk out because I was still waiting for someone to care enough to stop me. The void in my life where my parents belonged still haunted me. It ached like an infected wound. And while some people would have gone to therapy to heal it, I had no intention of ever going to therapy again. The word made me sick. It sounded stupid and naive. So instead of struggling to understand what my parents had done to me, I tried to heal that festering wound with love, just like Jennifer tried to heal it with pills and heroin. But now, even after talking about our relationship, when I asked her about her drug abuse, she always avoided the question.

"I can't talk about it yet," she told me. "Not until I figure out what I'm going to do."

A week later, in the beginning of August, Jennifer called to say she had gotten me an early birthday present. She drove out the next morning and we spent the day walking around the museum before going to get ice cream. When I asked about the gift, she sat back in her chair and crossed her legs and shoveled a tiny plastic spoonful of frosting into her mouth.

"Not yet," she said. "I want it to be a surprise for Robert too."

Jennifer called him when we got home. They spoke for a few minutes and she hung up and said that he and Julie had invited us over for dinner. We arrived to find them sitting in the shade on the back porch, grilling burgers while the kids played in the backyard. Paul scurried up to Jennifer and whispered something. She knelt to listen to him and he took her hand and spent the rest of the afternoon leading her around the house just so he could be near her. She seemed so happy, trailing him from place to place and smiling at me throughout dinner, like it was the greatest day of her life.

We finished dessert and then Julie said good night and corralled the kids off to bed. Jennifer and I followed Robert to his study. He closed the door behind us and sat at his desk. He was lighting his pipe when Jennifer reached for my hand.

"I'm going to a rehab clinic next week," she said. "It's in Arizona."

I turned and stared at her. She watched me for a long time, smiling and searching my eyes. I tried to speak. Then I began to laugh and burst into tears. I stood and held her as she leaned in to me.

"I'm tired," she said. "I want to get married. I don't want to be like this anymore."

Robert shuffled out from behind his desk and wrapped his arms around us. He was shorter than Jennifer and his gray hair was longer and more disheveled than in years past. He gave us a final squeeze and we all laughed and wiped our eyes and sat down. An hour later he walked us to the front door. The house was dark and quiet. We stood in the entryway between Julie's piano and the dining room and whispered good night.

"Thanks for everything you've done for me," Jennifer said to him.

Robert took both her hands and squeezed them. "You're welcome, daughter soon-to-be."

Jennifer and I went back to my apartment and I dug through the kitchen to find a bottle of wine we'd saved for a special occasion. I didn't know anything about wine when I bought it, except that it was expensive enough to put a smile on her face.

"You're not allowed to propose tonight, not until I get back," she said. "You promised."

She uncorked the bottle and set it on the living room floor. We sat facing each other with our legs crossed and then raised our glasses like two kids playing house.

"To my wife-to-be," I said.

We each took a sip and set down our glasses. Then I pushed Jennifer onto her back and kissed her. One of my legs grazed the bottle and a long crimson ribbon of wine streamed across the gray carpet. I jumped to my feet and grabbed the bottle. It was already half empty.

Jennifer knelt over the pool of wine and pushed her fingers into the soggy carpet.

"Oops," she said.

I crawled toward her as she stretched out on the floor between my arms. I kissed her forehead and stared into her eyes. We didn't speak for a long time.

"I sure love you," I said.

She leaned up and gave me a kiss. "I know you do."

Months before I met Jennifer, I began shopping for a house near the Andrewses. My bank preapproved a mortgage and gave me six months to find a place, but I stopped searching after a couple of weeks. The idea of buying a house scared me. I was only twenty-three, and I was still being sued by the doctors. My legal bills had exhausted nearly all of my savings. I wasn't even sure I wanted to settle down. Then I met Jennifer.

We had been dating for nearly four months when I found our house resting on a rural three-acre hilltop overlooking a lake. Its red clay tile roof and brick walls and low eaves made it look like a horse ranch in a Western film. The former owners were animal lovers and had used the living room as an aviary, so I hired a contractor to rebuild the interior. He said the work would take two months. And now that Jennifer was about to leave, it was almost done.

A few days before her flight, we tossed a six-pack of Shiner Bock into the back of my car and drove to the house to see the progress. We sat on the porch swing on the back patio and talked and sipped our beers while the sun nestled to sleep in the tall grass. The air smelled of fresh paint and sawdust. We sat in silence for a long time, swaying and listening to the crickets and the grass in the breeze. Jennifer straightened her legs and pushed the porch swing and then tipped back her head and finished her beer. Then she walked to the edge of the patio and pitched the bottle into the weeds. The brown longneck hummed a long, wavering note as it pinwheeled through the air.

Jennifer leaned against a post under the porch and stared at the grass.

"Let's get married in Rome," she said.

"Rome? Like Rome, Italy?"

She nodded without looking at me. "Sure. Let's elope."

"Well, Robert and your mom already know, so it's not really eloping."

"You think you'll ever tell your other family?" she asked.

It had been two years since I'd spoken to my mom; when she told me that Linda had given birth to my sister Emily. My other sister, Adrienne, was a stranger now. I couldn't recall the last time I'd spoken to her. And the last time I'd spoken to my dad, I was still in the hospital. I had just turned sixteen. I was twenty-three now.

I shrugged even though Jennifer wasn't looking at me. "I don't know."

The sun had set and the sky behind Jennifer was the same dark blue as the open ocean. I gazed at her standing at the edge of the patio in her short summer dress, with her long hair and pretty legs and dusty bare feet. The image of her made my heart race.

"You're still the most beautiful woman I've ever seen," I said.

She looked at me over her shoulder. "What about when I'm old and gray?"

"Then I'll be old and gray with you."

She turned to look through the windows behind me and into the living room, at the new recessed lights and bare concrete floor and dust and drywall.

"I wonder if we'll still be living here," she said. She sat next to me and stared at the weeds for a while. "I'll be at the clinic for a couple of weeks. You should just meet me at the airport when I get back. We can buy our rings in Rome and get married and then celebrate your birthday there."

I pushed the porch swing and put my arm around her shoulder. A single star winked from under the eaves of the patio.

Jennifer turned to look at the living room again. "The bathroom doesn't work yet, right?"

I shook my head.

"Can we go home?" she said. "My stomach's bugging me again."

We went back to my apartment and crawled into bed. I rubbed her back while she tried to fall asleep. She said her stomach trouble was from years of anxiety and drugs, and that it had gotten worse after agreeing to go to the clinic. It was the middle of the night when she rolled over and looked at me.

"I know the clinic's not the same as the hospital," she said. "But I'm still scared."

I got out of bed and pulled on some shorts. "I know what'll help you sleep."

Rollerblading had always been Jennifer's cure for insomnia. I fetched her skates out of her car and we wandered around my apartment complex as she traced long arcs through the darkness. She would fly around the building and pass me and then circle back, smiling while I pulled her along like a kid on ice skates. It was after three in the morning when we got back into bed. Five minutes later she was asleep.

We woke up late the next day. I took Tundra for a walk while Jennifer showered and packed her things. The morning was hot and cloudy and my clothes were damp with sweat by the time I returned. Jennifer was drying her hair in front of the mirror, so I sat on my bed and watched her.

"You'll be at the clinic the day after tomorrow, right?"

She nodded and rubbed a dollop of lotion between her hands before combing her fingers through her hair. "I need to stop by my place and pack before I go to my parents' house. It'll be safer to leave my car there while I'm gone."

The reality of her leaving suddenly settled on my chest like a stone. I pictured her tied up and locked in a hospital, like the one in my mind, with its clicking doors and screens on the windows. I didn't want her to go. I almost asked her not to. Jennifer looked at me in the mirror and smiled.

"I called the clinic last week," she said. "The lady I talked to was really nice. She told me they don't use restraints or anything like that. And we're allowed to go outside."

If anyone had a reason to hate therapy, it was Jennifer. She had been locked in the hospital for two years and been tied to a bed. And now here she was trying to calm me down because I was more afraid than she was.

She sat next to me on the bed and held my hand.

"I'll be back soon," she said. "I'll call you while I'm there. If they don't let me out, you and Robert can come rescue me."

Tundra trailed us downstairs. Jennifer knelt and kissed her forehead.

"I'll miss you, Tun. I'll see you when I get back."

I followed Jennifer to her car and opened the driver's door. She set her Rollerblades on the floorboard behind the seat. I laid her bags next to them.

"A few more weeks and we'll be in Rome," I said.

I wrapped my arms around her waist and kissed her neck. Her hair smelled like lotion and perfume.

"I love you," I said.

"I know you do, darling. I love you too."

I walked to the porch and stood next to Tundra. Then Jennifer backed out of her parking spot and blew me a kiss and mouthed the words we both knew so well.

"Alligator food."

15

Bast and the Black Easter Bunny

Jennifer called me from her parents' house that night. I sat on the floor near our wine stain while we watched an old black-and-white movie and talked about her leaving for the clinic and our going to Rome. It was after ten o'clock when she said she was going to take a bath.

"I'll call you back when I get into bed," she told me.

But she never called.

It was nearly two in the morning when I dialed her number. The line was busy, so I crawled into bed and set the phone on the sheets next to me and waited for her to call.

My room was hot the next morning. I had forgotten to close the blinds next to my bed and the bright August sun blazed between their narrow slats. I draped my arm across the sheets next to me and reached for Jennifer. Then I remembered she was at her parents' house. I glanced over to see the phone still resting on its side, then heard a knock on the front door.

Maybe she drove out to surprise me before she leaves.

I raced downstairs. The living room was dark. There was another knock as I reached for the door. Robert stood shadowed and backlit against the hot summer day. He had been crying. He stepped inside and stared at me as I closed the door and the room went dark again. I blinked until I could see him watching me. His eyes looked empty and tired.

"I'm sorry, Ban," he said. "I don't know how to say this." He wrapped his arms around me. "Jennifer died last night."

Everything went silent. Robert kept speaking but I couldn't hear him. I couldn't make sense of anything. I pulled away from him and slumped against the sloped banister of the staircase next to me, its painted wood cold and smooth. I pressed my forehead against it and closed my eyes.

"I knew she'd die before me," I said. "But not now. Not now."

I wandered into the living room and leaned against the wall, my body heavy, as if it had been filled with sand. My eyes settled on a familiar red stain on the floor.

The wine we spilled. We made love right there.

"I'm going to stay with you," Robert said. "I'm not going anywhere. I'm right here."

This isn't real, I thought. *She's leaving tomorrow.*

I imagined Jennifer dead, as if death looked like sleep. I almost began yelling at Robert. I wanted to tell him to go home. I wanted to believe he was lying and that all of this was some terrible joke. I imagined rewinding the entire night like a scene in a film, watching it all go backward until Jennifer was upstairs again, curled up in my bed in her ruffled socks. Huge, angry tears dripped down my face.

"She can't be dead," I said. "She's leaving tomorrow."

Robert didn't say anything.

"How did she die?" I asked.

"The coroner won't know for a few days."

I pushed the heels of my palms into my eyes.

I just want to go to sleep and wake up when this is over.

Robert used my phone to call a therapist. "You've met him at church a few times," he said. I let Tundra outside to go to the bathroom and then Robert drove me to an office I'd never seen before. Inside, there were curtains over the windows and the light was pale and yellow. The therapist looked familiar. He hardly spoke. I sat down and he just stared at me like I was some injured animal he had found on the side of the road, so I looked at Robert and talked about Jennifer, about how we used to walk around the museum and the botanical gardens and lie in bed and laugh together. After a while, I began repeating myself. Then I grew tired of speaking and stared at the windows and the trees behind the thin yellow curtains.

I woke up that night on the floor of my bedroom. I didn't know how I'd gotten there. Robert must have left and Tundra was curled up in front of me. "Jennifer's dead," I whispered in her ear. I began crying, then coughing and dry heaving. I tried to stop but I couldn't and I vomited on Tundra. I got to my feet and cleaned the floor and then filled the bathtub and washed her. She never struggled. She just watched me with her shining black eyes full of compassion. I had taken her out of the tub and started drying her when I thought of calling Jennifer. Then I remembered she was dead and I began crying again. I lay down on the carpet outside the bathroom and wept until I fell asleep.

Robert woke me the next morning. I was still on the floor. I didn't know how he had gotten inside. He said I had given him a key, but I didn't remember doing that. He held up a brown paper bag with something inside it.

"I brought you some food," he said.

He followed me downstairs and sat with me while I tried to eat. Then I went back to bed.

I woke up later that evening. I was staring at the night sky through the blinds next to my bed when I realized I hadn't washed my sheets in a week or two. *She was right here,* I thought, running my hands over them. *Her body touched these.* I buried my face in the soft flannel on her side of the bed. *I can still smell her.* I turned on the lights and searched my pillows and sheets for her hairs, then I coiled them inside a clear plastic bag and held them to the light. They looked like delicate strands of dark brown thread. I went through my closet and drawers and collected everything that belonged to her. Dresses. Lingerie. T-shirts she had taken from me. Each of them some mystical charm forever connected to her.

Then I remembered her answering machine. I began calling it over and over, listening to her voice and wondering how the woman and body that made that sound were gone now. Sometimes I would leave a message, and I would picture her sitting in some dark attic room in another world, where she would listen to me and smile as if she had never died at all.

I hung up the phone and dialed a random number. I don't know why. I knew Robert was probably asleep, and I didn't have many friends in Fort Worth. Someone answered before I could hang up, but they didn't speak. There was a long pause. Then a woman murmured.

"Hello?" she said.

I didn't answer.

"Hello?" she repeated. "Are you okay?"

"No," I said. "My fiancée died."

At first I thought she might say something. Then she began to cry.

"Oh my God, I'm so sorry," she said. Her voice was so kind. "I'm still here. I won't hang up. I'll stay on the phone as long as you need."

She listened while I talked about Jennifer and our time together. Sometimes I would fall quiet and she would speak after a moment and remind me she was still listening. Soon I drifted off to sleep. It was dark when I woke in the middle of the night. I didn't know how long I'd been out. Tundra was still next to me. I had dropped the phone, so I picked it up.

"Hello?" I said.

There was a rustling sound, then a sleepy voice. "I'm still here," the woman said.

"I'm so tired. I think I'm gonna try to sleep."

"I'll stay on the phone. You get some rest. Just say something or press some buttons if you need me."

The next thing I remember, someone was knocking on the front door. The sun was up. I had slept for hours.

"You awake, Ban?" Robert said from downstairs.

The phone lay next to me. I picked it up and spoke, but no one answered. I heard a radio in the background.

She probably went to work.

"Thanks," I said to the woman and the radio.

I hung up the phone and Tundra followed me downstairs. Robert was standing in the living room. He said the coroner had determined that Jennifer had died from cardiac arrhythmia.

"It wasn't an overdose," he told me. "He said her death was from years of drug abuse."

We were quiet for a long time.

"Her viewing's tonight," Robert said. "Her parents want you to have some time alone with her. I can drive you there."

"Can I put a few things in her casket? Will they bury them with her?"

"I'm sure they will," he said.

It was late afternoon when Robert drove us to the funeral home. We listened to Neil Young and I stared out the window at familiar meadows I had driven past so many times before. The world felt like a replica of a place I remembered, with fences and trees and a sky spread thin over something hollow and meaningless.

An hour later we parked in front of a brown brick building. I was following Robert toward the entrance when I stopped in the middle of the parking lot and stared at the fields of gravestones.

Jennifer's parents were standing in the foyer of the chapel. Her dad shook my hand. Her mom, Cecilia, gave me a hug.

"Take as much time as you need to say goodbye," she said. She gestured toward a small room. I could see Jennifer lying in a casket at the far end. I was too empty and tired to feel anything anymore. I just wanted to be near her.

Robert said something and then handed me the bag I had brought. Inside it were the few items I wanted to bury with her. Cecilia recognized one of them, a soft black Easter Bunny with a pink yarn nose. Jennifer had left it at my apartment before leaving for the last time. She said he wouldn't be happy at the clinic.

"It was always on her bed when she stayed with us," Cecilia said. "She slept with it every night. I know she'd love to have it with her."

Robert put his hand on my shoulder and guided me toward the room. "I love you, son," he said. "I'll be right outside if you need me."

Jennifer rested in an open casket lined with white satin and lace. She had been clothed in one of her favorite dresses. Her dark hair trailed over her shoulders and her eyes were closed, and most of her freckles had been covered in makeup. Beneath it, her skin was ashen. Someone had made her look a little too cheerful, but I was grateful to them for caring for her. She was almost smiling, as if imagining herself in a beautiful place. I thought of touching her, but it didn't seem right.

I knelt and folded my arms on the edge of her casket and gazed at her. My body felt brittle and hollow. I went to stroke her hair and something inside me opened and wave after wave of grief spilled out. I wept and leaned over her body, running my fingers through her hair as tears streamed down my face.

"Please come back," I cried. "Please. I can't do this without you. After making it this far and finally finding you. This wasn't supposed to happen. It wasn't supposed to be this way." I bent down and kissed her forehead, her skin waxy and cold against my lips. "God, Jennifer. I can't keep going without you. I can't keep doing this anymore."

I knelt next to her and wept for a long time. I wanted to go to sleep. I was so tired. I began banging my forehead on the edge of her casket. Then I imagined screaming and shaking her to life until she woke up and told me everything would be okay, like she had so many times before.

But it's not okay this time. She's dead now. The hospital killed her. It killed Kevin, too. And now it's going to kill me.

I wiped my face on my sleeve, then opened the bag that held her Easter Bunny and a letter I'd written the night she died. Lying in the bottom of the paper sack was a small black effigy of the Egyptian goddess Bast.

I'd given it to Jennifer when we first met. The figurine's feline gaze stared up at me from the darkness, its eyes offering some kind of unspoken vow to watch over her in the afterlife.

I rested the items in Jennifer's arms. The cheerful Easter Bunny looked strange next to her. I stood and stared at her, trying to memorize every detail for the last time. Then I leaned over her casket and kissed her cold lips.

"I love you, darling," I said. "I'll see you soon."

I didn't sleep the night before Jennifer's funeral. I wandered around my apartment, hostage to a body thirsty and hungry and unwilling to eat. It was inconsolable and wept until I'd nearly vomit. It forced me out of bed to urinate when I didn't want to get up. Then I'd crawl back between the covers and stare out the window and watch the sky turn from black to deep blue to aquamarine until Robert called to say he was coming to pick me up.

I pulled on my suit and shook some kibble into Tundra's bowl and then waited outside. Beads of sweat began trickling down my chest as the sun bore down on my brown wool blazer.

I looked down at my body.

I have to keep drinking water to keep this thing alive.

Robert drove us to the funeral while I stared out the window. The heat and humidity outside the car made the world seem hostile. Jennifer's family was so kind when we arrived. Cecilia walked over and gave me a hug while I stood next to Robert.

"You and Jennifer were as good as married," she said to me. "You're family now. You're gonna sit with us."

I was barely conscious for the funeral. I sat in the front row next to Jennifer's parents and brother while people filed past us and cried and hugged me and said they were sorry. Then a chaplain approached Jennifer's casket and everyone fell silent. He spoke for a while, standing there in his black suit and clerical collar like a man from a country that never saw sunlight. He offered a prayer and I stood with Jennifer's family and set a dozen white roses on top of her casket. I didn't know what to say. My mind and body felt empty. I thought for a while until some words came out.

"I brought your favorite flowers, darling. I love you. I'll always love you."

A group of men began lowering Jennifer's casket into the ground, so I stood by her grave with her family while more people cried and said they were sorry. Then Robert drove me home.

The funeral provided some closure, but I felt empty afterward. I'd been left with a body that needed sleep and nourishment, even though the rest of me had died. I wasted the next week playing computer games until I fell asleep at my desk. Then I'd wander upstairs and get into bed with one of Jennifer's dresses and pretend I was holding her until I drifted off to sleep.

But there were other things in my life I couldn't ignore. I had a dog that required food and water and companionship, and I was still being sued by the doctors. I also needed to move into the house I'd bought for me and my dead fiancée.

I began packing a few days before the house was ready. I wandered around my apartment and put things into boxes in no particular order. I placed all of Jennifer's belongings into three or four boxes and labeled them. The contents were a strange snapshot of our time together. Everything from clothing and books to half-burned candles and the empty bottle of wine we had spilled on the floor.

I was packing up the kitchen when Robert called. He said the contractor working on my house had been trying to reach me, but I hadn't answered the phone.

"They're putting in the carpet tomorrow," Robert said. "You'll be able to move in once they're done. Let's drive out this afternoon and take a look."

It was dusk when we pulled into the long gravel driveway, its stones rattling beneath the car as Robert stopped in front of the house. The living room lights had been left on and the house looked quiet and empty.

The last time I was here was with Jennifer.

I unlocked the front door and Robert and I stepped inside. The smell of fresh paint filled the house. The bare concrete floors had been lined with wooden carpet strips covered in tacks, and the wood-slatted vaulted ceiling had been painted white. Tall wooden bookshelves bordered a rock fireplace on the far wall. The house was bright and beautiful and radiated hope for a future that only seemed stupid and painful now.

I peered through the windows of the living room at the patio outside. The porch swing hung there, motionless and quiet. I thought of Jennifer sitting there and I walked toward the back door of the house. Robert followed me as I stepped onto the patio.

"Jennifer and I used to sit out here and talk. Sometimes we'd bring a couple . . ." I stopped midstride and stared at the tall grass. "Her bottle."

I bolted into the yard as I recalled the oscillating hum of the bottle cartwheeling through the air. The grass was as high as my chest. I stomped through the dry blades, using my arms to sweep them aside. By the time I'd made it ten feet into the yard, I was covered in foxtails.

"Please be here," I said. "It can't be gone."

"Ban . . . ?"

Robert probably thinks I've lost my fucking mind.

"I'm looking for her beer bottle!" I yelled. "She threw it out here last week!"

I found it lying on its side with the label facing the ground. It looked like a sacred relic resting there in the grass, last touched by her and then almost forgotten. I held it up for Robert to see as I turned for the house. It was the first time I had smiled in a week.

"That was Jennifer's, huh?" he said.

"She threw it out there the last time we were here. I can't believe I found it."

"I can. You should have seen yourself. You looked like a whirling dervish."

We had stepped back into the house when I noticed a dark gray patch on the living room floor. The workmen had filled an old electrical outlet. I knelt and touched it. The concrete was still soft.

I pulled my keys out of my pocket and looked at Robert and his face lit up in a grin. I sat on the floor and set Jennifer's beer bottle next to me. Then I said the words aloud as I carved them into the wet concrete with one of my keys.

"I. Love. Jennifer."

Robert put his hand on my shoulder. "She lives here now, like a vestal flame in a temple. She'll tend to this place and care for you."

He stepped back and offered me his hands. I took them and got to my feet as he lowered his head in prayer.

"Lord, bless this house with happiness and peace. Make it a home not just for Banning but for Jennifer as well. Guide him through this terrible time, and help him find the patience and courage to look ahead and see the years of happiness beyond this moment."

Robert closed his benediction and gave my hands a final squeeze before letting them go. He opened his eyes.

"Let's take a look at the rest of the house," he said. "Then we'll get you home. You look like a bale of hay."

Days later I stood with Robert in my empty apartment, staring at the wine stain on the living room floor. The door was open and the room was dark. Outlines in the gray carpet traced the placement of old furniture. Bright rectangles marked the walls where pictures once hung. I felt like the apartment, vacant and dusty and haunted by Jennifer's presence.

Robert asked about the stain, so I told him the story of the night we had knocked over the wine after saving it for a special occasion. His eyes filled with tears when I mentioned the clinic. In my grief I'd forgotten that he had lost a friend too, his "daughter soon-to-be."

I knelt and ran my fingers through the stain in the carpet. "I feel like I'm letting a part of her go."

"You are," he said. "You'll never be the same again. You lost part of yourself when you lost her."

Robert's words stirred my already fragile grief and I sat on the carpet and wept. He stood next to me for a moment before crouching by my side.

"I won't tell you everything will be okay," he said. "Nothing's okay. You lost your fiancée and your best friend. You're going to hurt and grieve for a long time. But I promise you, things will get better someday. I don't know how you've become the man you are after surviving the hospital, Ban. But if you can do that, you can do anything. And while you may not believe me now, I know there will come a day when you look back and realize that all this struggling was worth it."

16.

The House

I was twenty-four years old when I moved into the house that summer in 1995. I had a new family who loved me and an annuity that would support me for the rest of my life. My days were filled with free time and things to do. But none of it seemed to matter when all I wanted lay buried in an open field an hour away, in a small town called McKinney.

Before Jennifer's death, my suffering seemed temporary. I'd wake up every day and tell myself that whatever was hurting me would eventually come to an end. In the hospital, I compartmentalized my pain; I objectified it, as if my friends and I were simply characters in some terrible film. I'd grown so used to witnessing violence and trauma that my emotions didn't seem real anymore. I knew they were mine, and I could explain them, but my feelings seemed to exist somewhere else, somewhere deep inside me, in some little glass box that I could see but not open.

The only exceptions were rage and grief, and those emotions made me want to either tear myself apart or sleep for days.

But Jennifer's death was unlike anything I'd ever experienced. It felt like an enormous monolith that obscured the rest of my life. It didn't matter where I looked or how far I walked to circumvent it. She wasn't coming back, no matter how long I managed to survive.

Every afternoon I'd sit on the porch swing and stare at the grass and wonder how to feel grateful for a home I didn't want anymore. At first the house was empty, apart from the study, where my computer occupied a desk and a chair faced the monitor. The only other exception was the guest room, where I'd put the sleigh bed that Jennifer and I had shared. Its mattress and wooden frame seemed sacred with her gone, so I left them untouched and unmade. Instead, I slept next to Tundra on a pile of blankets on the floor in the master bedroom until Jennifer's new bed arrived.

Weeks before she died, we decided to shop for furniture for the house. I wanted a coffee table for the living room. She wanted sofas and a bed. We walked through half a dozen showrooms before we managed to agree on a lamp.

"We should each get one item the other can't veto," she said. "So if you find something you really love, then I can't say no. Same goes for you. You can't veto my item."

I didn't think much of it, so I agreed. An hour later I found my coffee table. Jennifer sat on a neighboring sofa and kicked off her shoes and then propped her feet on the edge.

"It's too pointy," she said. "It hurts. A coffee table needs to be a good footrest, too."

I shrugged. "Then I want this to be my one item."

Jennifer jumped to her feet and pulled me through the showroom, her long black skirt sailing behind her like the Wicked Witch of the West. She stopped at the foot of a colossal king-size poster bed. Its four wooden spiral columns stood more than six feet tall. When I tried to reach for the price tag, she grabbed my hand and smiled.

"It's my one item," she said.

The bed was a floor model. It would take months to make and wouldn't be delivered until we got back from Rome.

And now she's gone.

It was October when the bed finally arrived. I walked around it after the movers left, wondering at the mystery of Jennifer leaving me a gift months after her death. I unpacked her dresses and hung them in the closet on her side of our his-and-hers bathroom. Then I organized her keepsakes on her counter, where half-burned candles and a Pez dispenser sat next to her postcards and pictures and a pile of her clothing.

Thanksgiving arrived and the days grew short. Bright holiday lights sprang to life on the houses in the neighborhood. Every evening after sunset, I'd wander down my gravel driveway to find my mailbox full of manila envelopes and court documents from my attorney, William. He would call every few weeks and patiently reexplain the doctors' lawsuit, but it never made any sense to me.

"How can they sue me for libel and defamation when I haven't talked to anyone?" I said. "I didn't even speak in front of Congress, but they're suing me anyway."

William seemed convinced the suit was frivolous, but after a year and a half of legal bills my savings were gone. All I had left were my monthly annuity payments, and they barely covered my mortgage and bills.

By December I'd muted the ringers on all my phones except the one in my study. My social life consisted of reluctantly playing in a band with three friends from high school a couple of times a month. Every week or two they would make the hour-long drive from Rockwall and spend a few hours playing music or dragging me out to lunch, where I'd stare at the table and talk about Jennifer until they drove me back home, past neighborhoods filled with Christmas lights and decorations and happy couples who still had each other.

My life began to slowly devolve into a tiny world centered around my computer. Most days I'd play games for ten or twenty hours at a time. I began going to the grocery store in the middle of the night so I wouldn't have to talk to anyone. Daylight became strange and unfamiliar. I piled my trash bags in the garage because carrying them a hundred feet down the driveway meant having to see the mailbox and its mouthful of manila envelopes. Most nights I stayed in my study and played games until sunrise. Then I'd wander off to my bedroom and brush my teeth and gaze at the altar I'd built to Jennifer and her belongings.

"Good night, my love," I'd say. Then I'd kiss her picture good night and crawl into bed, only to wake up and spend another day sitting in a chair for hours, just like I had so many years before.

Christmas Eve was Robert's birthday. He and Julie invited me to stay over for a few days, but I never returned their calls because I didn't want to leave my computer. It wasn't until I heard his voice that morning that

I remembered I wouldn't have a computer, or a house, or my memories of Jennifer, if it weren't for him, so I went to my room and packed a bag to stay for one night.

I missed his birthday dinner and arrived late after playing games all day. The house was dark when I pulled into the driveway, and I could see Robert through his office window. He looked old and tired, hunched in front of his computer like a wizard toiling away in some forgotten tower, and I stood there in the darkness, feeling guilty for not being strong enough to leave my house for someone who had done so much for me.

I let myself inside and walked into his office and set an unwrapped bottle of cognac on his desk. He sat facing away from me, focused on a computer game.

"Happy birthday, Pop."

He turned from his monitor and glanced at the bottle. "Let's have a drink and wrap some gifts," he said. He stood slowly and I followed him out of his office, watching him lumber down the hallway in his favorite red flannel nightgown. His disheveled gray hair hung in tendrils down his neck.

I stepped into the kitchen to find the table covered in rolls of wrapping paper and boxes full of ribbons and decorations. Scraps of paper and tape covered half the room.

"Holy shit," I said. "I knew you loved Christmas, but . . ."

He pulled the cork on the bottle and poured two glasses and then handed one of them to me before we clinked them together and sat at the table.

"I didn't always feel that way," he said. "When I was a kid, my brother used to give me one sock for my birthday and the other for Christmas."

A smile crossed his face and then faded away. "How's my oldest and newest son?"

"Worried about the lawsuit."

The moment the words left my mouth, I wished I hadn't said them. Robert deflated in his chair. I'd been so absorbed in my own life that I'd forgotten the doctors were suing him too.

"They don't have a case," he said. "They're just trying to punish us. But there's not much we can do until the suit gets dismissed."

"But why's it taking so long? It's been like . . ."

"It's been a year and half," he said, gazing at his glass. "Putting all your money in the annuity is one of the best decisions you ever made. They can't go after it. Sean and I are going to have to pay out of our pockets, and we don't have a hundred thousand dollars lying around."

I shrank into my chair. "A hundred thousand dollars?"

"I'm sorry, Ban. I shouldn't have said that. There's a lot that can happen in the meantime. We can even sue to get our legal fees back when it's all over. It's not time to worry yet."

He stood and ruffled my hair on his way to the kitchen. The bottle of cognac gurgled as he poured himself another drink.

"I was just thinking out loud," he said. "Let's not worry about it tonight. It's my birthday."

It had been three years since I'd walked into Robert's office to find him sitting behind a desk piled high with papers and document boxes, when he still had salt-and-pepper hair and red cheeks and an easy laugh. Back then he talked about being an attorney like he had been recruited to help save the world. But this time he couldn't rescue us from the doctors, because Robert wasn't a savior anymore. This time he was one of the victims.

That night was Robert's forty-second birthday, but he looked sixty years old, leaning on the counter like some washed-up superhero staring at a half-empty bottle of cognac. I imagined walking into the kitchen and holding him and telling him everything would be okay, that we were in this together, like he'd always done for me. But I didn't believe it. Nothing was going to be okay. Jennifer was dead and the doctors were going to ruin what was left of my life. So I looked away and sat back in my chair and stayed quiet, as if I'd never left the hospital at all.

For months I hid from the world, driven by fear and anxiety to spend my days alone. I began canceling rehearsals, until my three friends from high school eventually stopped coming to see me, and my half-hearted commitment to the band faded away. Every time I heard a car pull into my gravel driveway, I'd crouch on the floor and peer under the blinds with my heart pounding in my throat. My house slowly disappeared behind a wall of weeds. The city sent an old man on a tractor to cut them down, and I hid in my bedroom until he left. When I went outside later that night, I discovered someone had purchased the lot next door and begun building a house about sixty yards away.

Other than my monthly trips to the grocery store or the occasional visit to see Robert, Julie, and the kids, my only time away from the house was spent at Jennifer's grave. I'd wait until nighttime and go to the store and buy a dozen white roses. Then I'd drive to the funeral home and wander through the moonlight before coming to a stop at the low mound of bare earth where Jennifer slept. I'd lie in the grass next to her grave and gaze through the ground, talking to her while I imagined her looking up at me and smiling, her arms still cradling her Easter Bunny and her figurine of Bast.

What would have been Jennifer's twenty-fifth birthday arrived in late December of 1996. I called her mom, Cecilia, the day before and we agreed to meet at Jennifer's grave. She showed up a few minutes after me and she knelt quietly and arranged her flowers next to my dozen white roses. She was meticulous, like a woman braiding her daughter's hair, fussing with each flower until she was happy with them. Then, without saying a word, she stood and put her arm around me.

"Do you have time for lunch?" she asked.

"Sure. It's not like I have anything else to do."

I followed her to a Mexican restaurant near their house. A hostess seated us at a small table near the bar. Cecilia sat next to me instead of across the table.

"How often do you come out here to see Jennifer?" she asked. Her accent made her sound like a social worker from New Jersey.

"A couple of times a week," I said. "It depends. I always come out for our anniversary and her birthday. And holidays too, like Valentine's and Easter."

She patted my hand. "You're so sweet, Banning. I know how much you still love her, but you've got to move on. It's been a year and a half."

There wasn't anything to say, so I straightened my silverware.

"Are you dating anyone?" she asked.

I shook my head.

"Are you working?"

God, I hate that fucking question.

"No," I said.

"You should volunteer somewhere. Go walk some dogs. You'll meet a girl. Jennifer would want you to be happy."

I hated those words. I wanted to yell at her and storm out. I'd heard the same bullshit from other people, that Jennifer would want me to move on and find someone else, as if replacing her would magically cure my grief.

I sat through the rest of the meal and then went home and rearranged Jennifer's belongings in the bathroom. I dusted her pictures and her empty beer bottle, then organized the rest of her clothing in the closet. When I found one of our candles in the bottom of a box, I set it on the counter and made a ritual of lighting it whenever I thought of her. A week later all that remained was a burgundy pool of melted wax.

The next time I went to the store, I bought an entire box of candles.

Spring arrived and the weeds reclaimed the land around my house. Tundra eventually blazed a trail through them, and I'd sit on the porch swing and watch her wander around the yard, the tall grass rustling and shivering in her wake. After a while she would reappear and we would sit together on the warm concrete of the patio while I picked the burrs out of her long white fur.

One afternoon, just as I'd finished cleaning her, I heard the muted ringer of the phone next to my computer. I was expecting Robert to call, so I held the door for Tundra and then ran to my study.

"Hey, Banning," a barely familiar voice said. "It's Nathan."

The name evoked a memory of the last time I'd seen him, at Robert and Julie's house two years before. I remembered sitting in the study and watching him play a game.

"I figured I'd call and see what you're up to," he told me.

He said it as if no time had passed, like we were old friends. It had been so long since I wanted to see someone that I couldn't tell whether I was nervous or excited. I responded without thinking. "You should come over."

The doorbell rang an hour later. I paused my game and walked into the entryway and Nathan smiled at me through the window. He was only a few years younger than me, but his curly brown hair and blue eyes made him look like an enthusiastic fourteen-year-old.

I pulled open the door. "Hey, man."

He held a white paper bag in one hand and a matching soft drink cup in the other. The red *W* logo printed on them stirred a long-forgotten memory of sitting outside a restaurant with my dad when I was young.

"Where'd you get that?" I said.

He stared at me for a moment before glancing at the cup. "What? This?"

"That's from Wienerschnitzel."

"Uh . . . yeah."

"Where the hell'd you get it?" I demanded.

"Well . . . from Wienerschnitzel. They just opened one by my house."

"Holy shit! We have to go."

He burst into laughter. "Right now?"

"Yeah, man. I'll drive. Be right back."

Nathan stood waiting on the porch while I disappeared into my study. I grabbed my keys and wallet and rushed outside and then locked the door and left him laughing in the driveway. I pulled up a moment later and he hopped in with his drink and bag of food. He looked around the car, his eyes wide in disbelief.

"Dude. You drive a Range Rover."

"Yeah, it's a long story."

"Is it okay to have food in here? I don't want to spill anything. It looks brand-new."

"Yeah, don't worry about it," I said. "It's cool."

We drove for half an hour, laughing and talking and listening to music. He never asked where I worked or why I lived by myself in a huge house surrounded by weeds. He never asked how I managed to buy a Range Rover. He'd finished his food by the time we arrived at Wiener-schnitzel, but he ordered one more hot dog anyway, as if it were important to share a meal with a friend. He said he was studying acting and that he'd always lived in Fort Worth and his parents were still married. I told him I'd grown up in California and that my parents had gotten divorced. I didn't elaborate. We were halfway through lunch when I remembered meeting his mom at church, when Robert introduced us and told me she'd worked on the lawsuit and read my chart. But if Nathan knew anything about it, he never said a word.

It was early afternoon when we got back to the house. Nathan followed me inside and sat on the floor of my study and petted Tundra while I played a game. Every time I asked if he wanted to do something else, he'd just smile and shake his head.

"I'm cool with sitting here and hanging out," he said.

We took a break and sat on the back porch with Tundra and shared a frozen pizza for dinner. Then I showed him around the house, making sure he wouldn't see Jennifer's bathroom counter and her collection of belongings. It was two in the morning when he said he needed to go home.

I paused whatever game I was playing and tried to think up an excuse for him to stay.

"You can crash here. There's a guest bedroom on this side of the house. No one's ever used it."

I thought of Jennifer. *He'd have to sleep in our old bed.*

"I've got class in the morning and rehearsal tomorrow," he said. "Thanks though."

He grabbed his keys and walked to the entryway, then knelt to pet Tundra before saying good night. From the front porch I could hear him get in his car and shut the door. I stood there for a long time, listening to him drive around the corner and down the hill, until all I could hear were the crickets and the wind.

Nathan's friendship undermined everything I'd come to believe about myself. He knew nothing about my life, but he still liked me. He wasn't a father figure or an advocate or someone who felt sorry for me. He wasn't an addict or a victim of neglect or abuse. He hadn't lost his fiancée or his parents. He was just a nice guy.

At first I wondered if we were actually friends. Not because I didn't like him but because I couldn't understand why he wanted to be my friend. Since the day I'd left the hospital, I'd surrounded myself with people from broken homes or abusive families, people who doubted themselves or hurt themselves or hated the world as much as I did. I loved those people because I understood their pain. The few exceptions, like

Doni and Zach, were friends who had a shared passion for something that felt meaningful. We made music. Our friendship had a purpose.

Nothing about my friendship with Nathan seemed to have a purpose. We watched movies and played games and sang in the car. We drove to 7-Eleven in the middle of the night and wandered the aisles, talking about whatever computer game we had left paused back at the house. Once, after we had spent nearly four days playing games, stopping only to sleep and use the restroom, Nathan finally went home and I called Robert and wondered aloud whether I was supposed to be doing more with my life.

"What's more important than being happy and spending time with friends?" he said. "You don't need to feel guilty for being happy, Ban. Not anymore."

But Nathan couldn't hang out every day. He had a life outside of our friendship. He had a girlfriend and went to school and lived with his parents. His mom, Sharon, had worked on my lawsuit, and I began wondering if she might tell him about the hospital. So every few days, whenever he came to visit, I'd mention something about the lawsuit and then wait to see what he would say. But he never seemed to know anything. The first time I told him I'd been in a hospital, he asked if I'd been in an accident.

"Not exactly," I said, watching him. "Didn't your mom tell you? She knows all about it."

He shrugged. "She told me she worked on your case, but she said it wasn't her story to tell."

My fear evaporated in those words. Not only because of what he had said but because of how he said it, without thinking, without reflection or pause. It hadn't even occurred to him to lie. That was part of what made Nathan so easy to like. He never spoke poorly of anyone. He never insulted anyone. When he and his girlfriend split up, he didn't even blame her. He just smiled and said things didn't work out. After the hospital and living with my mom, Nathan's kindness seemed supernatural.

Throughout the rest of the summer, Nathan would come over and drag me out of the house, beyond my wall of weeds and into a world filled with people and sunlight. We played D&D with his friends. He inspired me to study martial arts. He motivated me when I didn't want to leave the house. Sometimes we would go to a movie or sit down to lunch and I'd see something that reminded me of Jennifer or someone from the hospital, then I'd laugh or share a story and Nathan would just smile and listen, as if he loved those people as much as I did. I cherished those moments. Other than Jennifer, I hadn't had a close friend in years. I had forgotten the excitement of wanting to see someone, to look forward to something other than being alone. But of all the stories I shared with Nathan, I couldn't bring myself to tell him details about the hospital, or that the doctors were suing me and Robert. It seemed wrong to tell someone as good as Nathan about what had happened to me. I didn't want to scare him away.

17

You Don't Belong Here

y attorney, William, sat about twenty feet away, next to Robert and Sean at the front of a courtroom. His slender build, blue eyes, and chiseled features made him look like a movie star from the sixties. I imagined him speaking to me, his voice clear and calm in my mind.

You can do this, Banning. Just relax and think through your answers.

I was sitting on a witness stand and the doctor's attorney was questioning me. The doctors were all seated behind him. All of them, including Dr. Fisher, were watching me, their eyes still stoic like years before. The attorney kept yelling at me and shaking a handful of pages in the air. His voice was muted, like someone speaking on a telephone with their hand over the mouthpiece. I turned and glanced at the jury. *Why are they all staring at me?* I thought. *Did I say something wrong?* I couldn't remember what question had been asked or what I'd said. Everything seemed distant and hazy.

I looked at William again. He was leaning forward in his seat, watching me. The courtroom behind him was full of people and the walls were a soft pastel color, like the walls of my room in the hospital. The doctor's attorney sat down, then William stood up and asked me a few questions. I felt safer with him there, watching him walk back and forth while he calmly spoke to me. After a moment he said something to the judge. Then the judge dismissed me from the witness stand. I sat next to Sean again. He leaned over and whispered in my ear.

"Good job, buddy," he said.

I looked at Robert and he smiled at me. William patted my shoulder. He smelled like cologne. He leaned over and told me I'd done well, and I took a deep breath and sat back in my chair. My shirt was cold and sweaty. I turned to say something to Sean, but he was staring at the table, his long brown hair stuck to his forehead like he had fallen in a pool.

The judge adjourned the courtroom for an hour's recess. William leaned over and spoke to me and Sean.

"Remember, this is a pretrial procedure. We're just here to see what could happen in a real trial. With the right outcome, the doctors might drop the suit."

We went to lunch and waited for court to reconvene later that afternoon. When the judge asked the jury for their decision, everyone fell quiet and one of the jurors stood. They stated the verdict, then the judge restated it in legalese and adjourned the session for the day. None of it made any sense to me. Everyone in the gallery stood and began murmuring to one another as they filed out of the courtroom. The doctors and their attorney stayed behind.

William stood and spoke to Robert for a moment.

"What happened?" I asked. "Isn't there a guilty or not guilty or something?"

Robert began shoving some papers into his briefcase. "Doctors don't sue their patients," he said. "The jury knows that. The outcome isn't exactly what we'd hoped for, but the doctors didn't get any good news either."

I still didn't understand what had happened. I'd expected something different, something definitive, but nothing felt finished.

William walked over to the gallery and began speaking to someone. Robert finished packing up the rest of his things. I sat there watching him as he jammed documents and manila folders into his briefcase. I don't recall saying goodbye to Sean or William. I only remember following Robert out of the courtroom and wandering behind him as he stormed through the parking garage, his jaw clenched tight in anger.

The doctors' lawsuit was dismissed three weeks later, on April 13, 1998. The case had lasted more than three and a half years. I owed William and his firm over a hundred thousand dollars. After paying only a portion of the bill, I was left with a house I couldn't afford and tens of thousands of dollars of debt.

I began sleeping erratically. Some days I'd stay in bed for more than sixteen hours. Other days I didn't go to bed at all. When I finally received my first foreclosure notice, I had no choice but to file bankruptcy and negotiate a plan with the government to pay off my mortgage.

The lawsuit had taken an even greater toll on Robert, Julie, and the kids. They didn't have an annuity to insulate them from the financial burden of an enormous legal bill. Robert began calling me at strange hours.

"I'm tired, Ban," he said once. "I'm tired of everything. I'm broke. The doctors ruined me. I can't keep hiding like this. Everyone knows I'm gay, even Julie; they just pretend I'm not. I feel like I'm trapped in a life that's not even mine anymore."

I didn't know what to say. I wanted to help Robert. I wanted to tell Julie. Maybe she knew already, I wasn't sure. I knew they loved each other, but I didn't want to interfere in their relationship. It didn't seem right.

It was then that I started getting angry again. At first it was small things. I'd drop a fork or a pencil or get upset at a game, then a huge, gut-wrenching rage would come lashing out of me. I hadn't experienced that kind of anger since my years of drumming in high school. I felt aimless and undirected, furious at everything and nothing. It wasn't until I took my cordless phone outside and screamed while I hurled it at the brick wall of my house that I realized something was wrong. Normal people didn't destroy cordless phones for having intermittent static. Only people who had something wrong with them did things like that.

With the lawsuit and the bankruptcy behind me, Nathan's friendship was all that I had left. I'd call every day to see if he could come over, then I'd go outside and sit on the front porch until he pulled into the driveway. Anyone peering in the windows would have seen two overgrown teenagers wasting their time. But to me, Nathan was the best friend I'd ever had. So when he called to say that his parents were moving to Arkansas that summer, I felt like I'd won the lottery.

"Dude, you can live with me," I said.

"No I can't. I don't have any money for rent, and I'm still trying to find some acting gigs. I don't even have a job right now."

"Fuck rent," I said. "I don't need your money."

It was a lie. For weeks I'd been selling stuff at a pawn shop to help pay for groceries and food for Tundra, but that day I would have given anything to keep Nathan from moving away. His friendship was all I had left.

Nathan moved in sometime that June, and what began as a friendship turned into a summer vacation filled with video games and frozen pizza. By then I'd told him more about the hospital, about sitting chair and restraints and Sonia's bed in the hallway. I even admitted that I'd filed for bankruptcy because the doctors had sued me. But none of it scared him away. He'd just pause whatever game he was playing and listen to me.

"How could the doctors sue you after everything they've done?" he said.

I shrugged. "I don't know. It was some legal loophole or something."

He turned to look at me, his eyes wide in disbelief.

"No, I don't mean legally," he said, raising his voice. "I mean, how could they fucking do that? It's wrong. Period. They made you sit in a chair and they tied people to beds and then they sued you guys. How is that okay?"

I didn't know what to tell him. The lawsuit never made any sense to me either. So we went back to our routine of playing games and watching movies, until the day Jonathan called me.

Jonathan was an acquaintance I'd met online months before. We had spent hours playing games and talking about books and our lives and our pasts. The internet's veil of anonymity made it easier to confide in people. No one knew me. They didn't know about the hospital or the lawsuit or the weeds around my house. But real friendships grew out of some of those acquaintances, and Jonathan was one of them. The first time we spoke on the phone, I felt like I'd known him for years. He was an artist who lived on the road, following his welding mentor from one art fair to another. When he called to say he was in town, I offered to let him crash at the house. Nathan was incredulous when I told him.

"You've never even met this guy?" he said.

"No, but he's cool. We've talked on the phone for months."

He shook his head. "Well, I'm taking Tundra and locking my door tonight."

We made the ten-minute drive to the grocery store where Jonathan had told me to meet him. I didn't know what he would look like, but when we pulled up to find a scruffy-looking guy pointing a camera at a large sculpture of a bull, I knew it was him. I rolled down Nathan's passenger window and Jonathan walked toward us. Other than his huge smile and his camera, he looked like he had been shipwrecked on an island for a few years.

"That sculpture's fucking amazing," he said, tossing his thumb over his shoulder. "I can't believe they put that thing in front of some shitty grocery store in the middle of bumfuck nowhere." He patted the side of my car. "Dude, you really do drive a Range Rover. Get the fuck out, man. Gimme a hug."

Nathan and I stepped out of the car. I stood barefoot on the concrete still warm from the summer day. Jonathan gave me a bear hug after refusing a handshake.

"I'm driving that pile of shit over there," he said, pointing at a run-down silver van speckled with rust. "Let's see if it can make it to your house. I'll follow you."

It was after midnight by the time Jonathan finally got out of the shower. I was sitting in the guest room, watching Nathan play a game, when Jonathan walked into the room.

"Don't you guys do anything other than play fucking video games?"

"Don't trash games, man," I said. "That's how we met."

"I like games, dude. Games are great. But so is bourbon, and I'm not drinking it for fucking breakfast. All things in moderation, right?"

Whatever reservations Nathan had about Jonathan staying the night dissipated in our laughter. Jonathan just stood there staring at us, wondering why we were laughing about wasting our lives.

The three of us sat on the back porch with Tundra while Jonathan shared stories about life on the road. It was hard to imagine living in a van and wandering from place to place, but there was something alluring about it. Jonathan had almost nothing, yet he seemed like one of the happiest people I'd ever met. He didn't care about having a plan or controlling his life. He wanted to learn and experience things and see the world. Freedom seemed to be all that mattered to him. And not just freedom to go somewhere or do what he wanted but freedom from worry and fear. I'd never heard someone talk about life like every day was an adventure, even when things went wrong.

It was probably three in the morning by the time we decided to go to bed. I was setting out some sheets and a blanket for Jonathan when he came out of the kitchen.

"Thanks again for letting me crash here," he said. "I'll have to repay the favor someday. I've gotta get you out of this house before you get a case of rickets."

I nodded. "It'd be cool to come visit you somewhere."

"I'm gonna hold you to that, man. You need to get out of this fucking state. You don't belong here." He turned for the living room and waved good night over his shoulder.

I knew he was right, although I never would have admitted it to him. Texas had never felt like a home. I'd been sent here, only to live through the worst years of my life. But as with the hospital, I had grown accustomed to it. It was predictable and familiar. It didn't matter that I was miserable; I wasn't about to walk away from Jennifer's grave and everything I'd known for the last fifteen years so I could slowly disintegrate in some strange and unfamiliar place.

That night I went to bed with the window open. I listened to the crickets while the morning sky turned from black to dark blue. I thought of Jonathan's stories about traveling and the world, and how my dad used to take me hiking and sailing when I was a child, when we used to sit together under trees and watch hawks wheel overhead. I thought of him letting me shift gears in his little red sports car, and going swimming at night, and how he'd wrap me in a towel and hold me while I was shivering. It had been a long time since I'd missed my dad. I wondered if I'd ever see him again, or if I'd just stay in Texas and play video games with my friend in a house hidden behind a wall of weeds.

It was a beautiful autumn evening, months after Jonathan's visit, when Nathan told me he was moving away.

"A good friend of mine moved to the Bay Area few years ago," he said. "A couple of friends of his just got a job at a software company.

They're still hiring. He said I can crash at his place for a while until I get a job."

I panicked. I didn't want him to go. I felt like a kid again, alone at the airport.

"Dude, you can't," I said. "Why would you work at a software company? You're an actor. How are you going to find acting gigs when you're stuck in a cubicle all day?"

For days I tried to convince him not to leave, secretly hoping his plans would fall through or that he would change his mind. Soon I realized that being a good friend meant caring more about Nathan's happiness than my own, so the morning he left I did my best to smile while we stood in the sunlight and said goodbye. Then he backed down the gravel driveway and drove away, honking as he headed around the corner and down the hill and off to California.

Except for my trips to the pawn shop or the grocery store, or a rare visit to see Robert, Julie, and the kids, most of my excursions out of the house ended when Nathan moved away. His absence left a gaping hole in my life. And without the courage to fill it with a job or school or something meaningful, I returned to my computer and my late-night trips to Jennifer's grave.

Then, weeks later, Robert called me in tears.

"I can't do it anymore, Ban," he said. "I can't keep living like this. I told Julie everything. She knows I'm gay. Everyone at church knows it now too."

I was terrified. He sounded suicidal. All I could think about were all the times he had propped me up and kept me going. I wanted to do the same for him.

"You still have me, Pop. I'm not going anywhere," I said.

"That's nice of you to say, but the doctors ruined me. I'm broke now. I can't even pay my cell phone bill. I had to borrow money. I don't have anything left."

"You're not going to do anything stupid, are you?"

"No, Ban. I'm moving to Austin. I have a friend down there that I can stay with for a while. Maybe I can start over there."

It was after midnight when we hung up. He promised he would call me when he settled in Austin. When I woke the next day, I thought of calling Julie and the kids, but I didn't know what to say to them. I'd hidden Robert's secret from them for years. So I avoided them, along with everything else in my life.

18

Like Oil and Pennies

I t was a winter afternoon when the rattling of a diesel engine woke me. I'd started sleeping with the covers over my head, and I opened my eyes to see a small patch of late-day sunlight where I'd made a hole so I could breathe. The truck's engine pitched high and loud as it headed up the hill around the corner from my house. Every weekday, around the same time, the UPS driver came racing through the neighborhood, the truck rumbling around like a big metal barrel on wheels. No one ever sent me anything, so I'd gotten to know the engine's exact pitch and volume as the driver passed my house. But that day the truck turned into my driveway, and the gravel popped and crunched as it came to a stop.

God, I hate that fucking sound.

I pictured the truck in my mind's eye, parked outside my bedroom, as if the walls of my house didn't exist. I could hear the driver stomping around inside the cab. I hated them for being there, for invading the only place I had left to hide. When they finally stepped down onto the gravel and walked past my window, a hot, sulfuric rage began to burn inside of me.

The driver rang the doorbell. I wanted to scream at them. I wanted to hurt them for being there. I imagined running to the kitchen and grabbing a knife and jabbing it into their eyes. I pulled the covers around me and waited until the truck clamored back to life and then faded away. Then I crawled out of bed and opened the front door to find a box waiting on the front porch. The names and addresses were written in familiar handwriting. I leaned forward to read them and stared at the return address for a moment.

It's from Dad.

I nudged the box with my foot and it scuffed across the concrete. Despite being big enough to hold several books, it weighed almost nothing. I carried it inside and set it on the floor in the entryway and stared at it for a while.

It's not my birthday, I thought. *Is there some holiday I'm forgetting? Did something happen? Is Dad okay?*

I peeled off the tape to find a framed picture inside. A piece of cardboard covered the front. For a moment I thought Dad might have sent me a family portrait featuring him and Linda and Henry and my new sister, Emily, but the frame looked familiar. My heart began to race as I peeled off the rest of the tape and lifted the cardboard covering the picture.

Underneath it lay a needlepointed portrait of my nine-year-old face. My dad had made it when we were still a family, then hung it in our living room next to the one he had made for my sister Adrienne. I'd seen

the portrait thousands of times. Now, twenty years later, with its burgundy background and blue-gray dots, it looked like some arts and
crafts project from a garage sale. I sat on the floor for half an hour, staring at my childish face grinning back at me from the past. I pitied that
kid now. He had no idea what was going to happen to him. If he had, he
would have just hung himself in high school.

I walked to my study and got the phone and dialed Robert's number.
We hadn't spoken since he had moved to Austin weeks before, but there
was no one else who really understood me. I felt guilty for always calling
him when I needed something.

He sounded happy when he answered. We talked for a couple of minutes and he said things had improved since he had moved to Austin. He
was renting an apartment and doing some legal work to pay the bills.
When he asked about me, I walked back into the entryway and told him
about the needlepoint. I could almost hear him smile over the phone.

"That's great news," he said.

"No, it's not. My dad probably found it in the attic and doesn't want
it anymore. He's getting rid of me."

"No, he's not, son. He's reaching out. He would've just thrown it away
if he didn't care, but he kept it all these years, and now he's sent it to
you. You should call him and thank him for sending it. It would mean
the world to him."

I set the picture back in the box and folded it closed.

"Maybe someday," I said. "Not today."

Robert fell quiet for a moment. "You can't keep waiting, Ban," he
said. "Remember, your dad's just as afraid of getting hurt as you are. If
you both keep waiting for the perfect time to reach out to one another,
it'll never happen. There is no perfect time. Trust me."

I went to bed early that night. It was cold and Tundra was curled up in front of me. The littlest spoon, Jennifer called her. After lying awake for hours, I went to my study and sat in the dark and stared at the needlepoint, my nine-year-old face beaming back at me like a missing kid on a milk carton. It reminded me of being a child, when I used to sit in front of the bathroom mirror and look at myself and imagine who I would be someday.

The sun had started to rise when I put the needlepoint back in its box and shoved it in a closet. I couldn't sleep and I was too tired to play a game, so I wandered the house, thinking about my dad and the needlepoint and why he had sent it to me after all these years. I didn't feel right that morning. I felt empty, like I had been cut open and hollowed out and whatever had been left inside me only made me feel sick and scared.

Years before, shortly after the doctors sued us, Robert took me and a friend from the hospital to meet a therapist in New York. Robert said we might need an expert witness. He promised it would only be one visit and that we would be safe. He sat outside the room while I told the doctor about the hospital and sitting chair, and Sonia and restraints. The doctor looked horrified. I'd never seen a psychiatrist actually react to something. I wondered if he had broken some kind of oath by getting upset. After a couple of hours, we wrapped up and he said, "Would you like to know what I think?"

"Are you allowed to tell me?" I asked. "Isn't that against the rules or something?"

The doctor smiled and shook his head. "You suffer from depression and PTSD, most likely as a result of some of your early experiences, especially your time in the hospital."

I was confused. "I thought soldiers got PTSD, like people who've been in combat."

"They can, yes," he said. "But so can many other people. PTSD is actually very common, and it's treatable. Not through medication but through therapy, through talking about your experiences."

I wanted to punch him in the face. I began laughing and he asked why.

"Therapy did this to me," I said.

He nodded and told me I would have to find someone I trusted, someone I could talk to about what happened in the hospital. I don't remember what else he said. I don't even remember saying goodbye. All I remember is walking out the front door of the hospital into the warm air and sunlight and thinking, *There's no way in hell I'll ever see another therapist again.*

Tundra was still curled up on the bed when I went back to my room and opened Jennifer's closet. A handful of her dresses hung in long, neat lines. They still smelled like her. I held one to my face and drew a breath. My favorite, a short black dress dotted with small white flowers, hung near the door. I took it off the hanger and held it at arm's length, imagining her standing with me in the closet and smiling, with her dark hair and hazel eyes and Cleopatra eyeliner.

I stepped out of the closet and then stopped when I saw myself in the mirror. I looked like a castaway—naked, skinny, and unshaven, holding some dress I had found on a beach somewhere, my wiry brown hair and beard as neglected as my yard. I ran my fingers over my ribs.

Yeah, that's me, I thought.

I walked back into the bedroom and unfurled Jennifer's dress on the floor as if I were clothing her ghost. She looked empty and incomplete, like a paper doll without limbs. "I'll be right back," I told her. I went to the closet and got a pair of her black stockings and a pair of her heels. I laid her stockings on the floor, one at a time, making sure to tuck each lace top underneath the hem of her skirt. Then I set her heels on the floor and put the feet of her stockings into them. Her hair and face and arms were missing, but they were buried an hour away, along with her Easter Bunny and Bast and the notes I'd put in her casket, so I sat on the floor and talked to what was left of her.

"I don't know what's wrong with me, love. It's been five years and you're still all I think about. I don't even care about being happy anymore. Sometimes I'd rather be dead than alive without you."

I was still sitting on the floor when I heard Tundra's nails clicking on the tile in the hallway. I turned around to see her staring at me. I felt self-conscious, like she had caught me doing something strange. I could tell she needed to go out, but I didn't want to leave Jennifer. Then Tundra sat and watched me.

"Goddamn it."

I pushed myself to my feet and then stormed through the living room with Tundra trotting happily behind me. I shoved open the door and stepped outside and she bolted into the yard and disappeared into the weeds. I was still naked, but I lived on three acres of land and could barely see the nearest house. The air was cool and felt nice, so I stood there watching the weeds shiver above Tundra while she roamed around the yard. One minute passed. Then two.

"Tundra!"

She stopped and the weeds fell silent. I pictured her looking in my direction, with her pointy white ears listening to me. Then the weeds began to rustle again and she returned to wandering around.

"Tundra! Goddamn it! Come on!"

She didn't stop this time. She just wandered farther away. I didn't want to be outside; I wanted to be with Jennifer. For a moment I thought about running out and grabbing Tundra and dragging her inside, but I was naked and the weeds were almost as tall as me. Then there was a loud rustle and she came running back onto the porch, grinning as if she were laughing at me. She was covered in foxtails.

"God-fucking-damn it. Now I have to clean all the burrs out of your hair." I yanked open the door. "Get the fuck inside!"

She looked at me for a moment. She had never seen me that angry. She knew something was wrong and I began shouting at her again and she ran inside. I chased her down the hallway and into the bedroom, where Jennifer's dress and stockings and heels lay on the floor like she had been disintegrated. Tundra darted under the bed and I lunged for her. Then she crawled out of reach and cowered against the back wall and stared at me with her eyes wide and her tail tucked between her legs, as if she were sorry for everything that had ever happened to me, for my parents and the hospital and Jennifer's death. But it was too late now. I didn't want sympathy. All I wanted was to unleash all the pain and fear and rage I'd buried inside of me.

I pointed at Tundra. "You're fucking dead."

I knew she would try to run, so I got up and closed the door. Then I crouched beside the bed to see her still huddled underneath. When I reached for her, she scurried out from under the bed. Then she stopped when she saw the door was closed and began crawling toward the wall. I grabbed the scruff of her neck and knelt on the floor and then pulled her face toward mine, almost daring her to growl or snap at me. Not because she had done anything wrong but because I hated myself and my life.

With Tundra still pinned to the floor, I raised my fist and willed myself to unleash all the pain and rage inside me, but my body refused to listen. Then a bright yellow puddle of urine began to form beneath Tundra. I let go of her and stared at it and then realized what I had done. I leaned forward and touched her. She began to shiver. A sickening wave of humiliation welled up inside me. I lay down and held her and wept, my arms lying in her warm pool of urine.

Then I saw Jennifer's dress. I felt like she had witnessed what I had done.

"God, Tundra. I'm sorry. I don't know what I'm doing. I can't live like this anymore."

Before I had finished saying the words, I remembered.

I have a gun.

I walked to the dresser beside my bed. Hidden in the back of one of the drawers was a pistol Robert had given me before Jennifer died. He had taken it from a client who had told him they were suicidal. It seemed like a terrible idea to give me a gun, but Robert had said he didn't want it at home and asked me to hold on to it for a while, so I'd taken it and hid it in the back of my dresser and forgotten about it. Until now.

I stood next to the bed and held the pistol. I didn't know much about guns. It seemed small and it was heavy, but something in that weight made me feel like I had found a solution to a problem. I lay down on my side with my back to the window, facing Jennifer's bathroom counter and her collection of belongings. I imagined putting the gun in my mouth and pulling the trigger and seeing Jennifer appear in front of me.

Then Tundra jumped onto the bed.

I began to shoo her away before realizing I didn't need to worry about getting dog urine on my sheets when I was about to kill myself, so I lay down again and put the barrel of the gun in my mouth and pointed it upward. The metal was cold and tasted like oil and pennies. Then Tundra curled up in front of me, where she always slept. The littlest spoon. I looked at her and imagined the sound of the gunshot. Her bright-black eyes wide and shocked. Her snowy white fur speckled with crimson dots. Her ears ringing. Her panic and confusion. I pictured her heartbroken and whining, lying next to my corpse for days until the UPS driver reported the smell.

Then, for some reason I still don't understand, my mind conjured the words of a friend I had met after high school, when I told her I thought the hospital had ruined me forever.

"You can't let the doctors win," she had said.

She was one of the first people I had ever told about the hospital. Her mom had committed suicide when she was young, and she always seemed to understand me when other people didn't. At the time, her comment sounded like bullshit. But now, lying on my bed with a gun in my mouth, I finally heard the truth in those words. Since my first night on unit B, the doctors had warned my parents that I would commit suicide. I had never even considered it before the hospital. But the idea haunted me, like a suggestion planted in my mind. And now here I was, about to fulfill the prediction of a small group of doctors who thought sitting in a chair and not going outside was a cure for depression. Suddenly that seemed even more sad than killing myself.

I crawled off the bed and put the gun back in my dresser. I felt light and euphoric. Tundra was still covered in foxtails and urine, so I carried her to the bathroom and gently set her in the tub. I have no memory of bathing her. Ten minutes later, she was running around the house, dripping wet and wagging her tail, smiling as if she knew that the worst of our lives was behind us now, and all that mattered was tomorrow.

19

You've Got to Let Me Go

few weeks later I sold my Range Rover. After putting most of the money toward my bankruptcy payments, I searched the newspaper for a car I could maintain on my own. Three thousand dollars later, I pulled into my gravel driveway behind the wheel of a rusty 1971 Ford Bronco with holes in the floorboard.

I'd never learned how to work on cars, so I began reading textbooks on basic maintenance. Every afternoon I'd go out to the garage and crawl under the hood with one of my grease-stained auto manuals and figure out how to replace the spark plugs or rebuild the carburetor. Then once the sun had started to set, I'd sit on the porch with Tundra and stare at my new car, recalling the day I'd signed the settlement agreement in Robert's office, when he handed me a calculator and asked me figure out the value of each day I'd been kept in the hospital. I could still remember gazing at those numbers and making a promise to do something with my life. But after spending the last few years hiding in a house with a ghost and a computer and a dog, I realized that being happy didn't mean avoiding more pain. I'm not even sure it required some tools or a broken-down car, because when I look back on those days now, my happiest memories aren't filled with images of my greasy auto manual or the underside of my Bronco—they're the moments I spent sitting outside with Tundra, listening to the crickets while I watched the sun set through the weeds on top of the hill next to my house.

Not long after I'd finished most of the repairs on my Bronco, my friend Jonathan called me. He had driven his rusty van to California and gotten a job in some place called Camp Mather, near Yosemite National Park. He was working as a cook and spent most of his free time fishing in the Tuolumne River. A twinge of jealousy shot through me.

"Damn," I said. "I'd love to be there. I really miss California."

He burst into laughter. "Then why the fuck are you still living in Texas?"

Those words sank into me like a rock in a pond. I didn't have an answer, so I made up an excuse.

"Tundra's getting kind of old. Moving would just stress her out," I said.

"Dude, she'd re-adjust faster than you. Not to mention, didn't Nathan move out here? He's probably just a few hours away."

The truth was the only two things keeping me in Texas were the house and Jennifer's grave. I didn't have a job and Robert had moved away. And now that I had filed bankruptcy, keeping the house seemed unlikely.

Jonathan lowered his voice. "Banning, your two best friends are out here in California, man. You've gotta move on. You're out of fucking excuses."

In retrospect, that was the moment I knew I would leave Texas someday. It had never been my home. I'd never wanted to live there. I didn't dislike Texas, but it had always felt like a prison, with its massive suburbs filled with painful memories. And while I wasn't ready to move to California yet, Jonathan's words and the image of him standing next to a river in Yosemite haunted me for months after that phone call.

Days later I dreamed of standing in a long hallway so narrow that my shoulders touched the walls. At the end of the corridor was a frosted-glass window filled with bright sunlight. The walls of the hallway were lined with dark wood embellished with squares, like rows of chocolate bars facing one another. A phone began to ring, so I turned my shoulders to the side and started shuffling down the hallway to answer it. I felt like I knew the place, even though I'd never seen it before.

The phone kept ringing. I wandered forward as it grew louder. The left side of the hallway was lined with wooden doors, one after the next. I remember thinking they were offices when I heard the phone begin to ring inside one of them. The office belonged to someone else, but the call seemed important, so I pushed the door open and walked inside.

Jennifer's clothing hung throughout the room, all of it neatly arranged on hangers. Her little black dress with white flowers. Her sweaters and skirts. Even the T-shirt she had taken from me to wear as a nightgown.

And the room smelled like her, as if she had just gotten dressed and walked out the door.

The phone rang again and I turned to see a black rotary telephone sitting on a small wooden table. I reached out to answer it, watching the hand in my dream, mine but not quite mine. The glossy receiver felt cold against my ear.

"Hi, love," Jennifer said.

A surge of emotion rushed through me. I tried to speak, but I was so overwhelmed that all I could say was "I love you. I love you. I love you," over and over and over.

She laughed softly. "I love you too," she said. "You don't need to cry anymore. Everything's okay now."

There was a realness in those words, as if she had whispered them in my ear. I remember thinking I needed to calm down and speak clearly, that she was close now and I didn't have much time.

"I've missed you so much," I said. "I still think of you every day."

She was quiet for a while. I could tell she was smiling when she spoke again.

"I've missed you too, sweetheart. But you can't keep holding on to me. You've got to let me go."

Then she hung up.

Less than a week after my dream, I put the house up for sale. The Realtor's sign appeared in the front yard a few days later and I walked to the end of the driveway and stared at it, wondering if I had made a mistake.

But when I turned around and looked at my house, with its red brick walls and clay tile roof and barely tamed weeds, instead of feeling fear or regret, I didn't seem to feel anything at all. I just didn't want to live there anymore.

The house sold three months later. Weeks before the sale closed, Nathan lost his job in San Francisco and needed a place to live. I'd never been so happy to see a friend file for unemployment. The day he arrived I knew I'd stay in Texas, at least until he moved back to California, so we rented an apartment a few miles away and spent the next couple of weeks packing up the few belongings I had decided to keep, including Jennifer's enormous king-size poster bed.

It was a hot summer day when Nathan and I stood together in the entryway and stared at the empty living room. The front door was open and a warm breeze drifted through the house.

"I still remember the first time I came here," he said, "when I was holding that Wienerschnitzel bag and you freaked out. I kept wondering why you lived in this huge place all by yourself."

Those words suddenly made me wonder why I had stayed for so long. I'd spent over a thousand days of my life playing games on my computer. It seemed unbelievable, all the things I could have done with that time. I could have sold the house and driven across the country and visited places I'd never seen. I could have learned to paint or write. I could have moved to a small town in some beautiful place and gotten a job at a nursery. Instead, I'd wasted years sitting in a chair facing a monitor instead of a wall. I'd always assumed I'd kept the house because it felt connected to Jennifer. But standing there with Nathan and staring at that empty house filled with nothing but broken dreams, I realized

I'd spent the last five years re-creating the hospital that had damaged me, that I'd hidden from the world because I'd never learned how to live in it. And now, for some mysterious reason, I wanted to be a part of it again.

I stood motionless and quiet, just a few feet away from Nathan. I wanted to say goodbye to the house, but I couldn't do it now, not with Nathan there, so I promised to come back later.

We made the fifteen-minute drive to our new apartment and un-loaded the truck and then ordered a pizza and watched a movie. Once the sun had started to set, I told Nathan I'd left something at the house and that I'd be back soon.

Texas is hot in the summer, even at night, and my Bronco didn't have air-conditioning. Even with the windows down, I was dripping with sweat by the time I pulled into my old gravel driveway. I shut off the ignition and peeled my legs off the vinyl seat and hopped out of the car. The house was dark and quiet.

This will be the last time I ever come here, I thought.

I went inside and walked to the far end of the living room, where Robert and I had once stood when we came to look at the house and I used my keys to write in the wet concrete. The words were covered up by the carpet now, but I knelt and traced them anyway, repeating them out loud, just as I had years before.

"I. Love. Jennifer."

I walked out onto the patio and sat in the porch swing and listened to the crickets and the wind. The day's last light was nothing but a milky blue line on the horizon. I imagined Jennifer in her summer dress, standing on the edge of the porch and staring at the first stars of dusk. I got up and walked to where she had once stood, then I knelt and kissed the concrete her feet once touched.

"I'll always love you," I said.

I went back inside and locked the front door and then got in my Bronco and cranked the ignition. I backed down the driveway until the car rolled into the street and the gravel fell silent. The engine rumbled quietly while I stopped to look at the house one last time.

She's not there anymore.

I shimmied the shifter into first gear and coaxed my old car forward, away from a house that never quite belonged to me and a life I had never wanted to live, not without Jennifer.

By the spring of 2001, Nathan had gotten a job at a movie theater near our apartment. I still had too much free time, so I bought a bike and began riding to Starbucks and reading books. I tried sitting inside at first, but after years of solitude the noise made it impossible to concentrate. Soon I found a quiet corner on the patio, where I began working my way through Pulitzer Prize winners and biographies. After a few weeks, baristas remembered my name and order. Then regulars started talking to me. The cardiologist from Canada who loved economics. The friendly English woman who shared my passion for sitting outside. Even the local Baptist minister who enjoyed discussing theology. I couldn't avoid making friends; other people made sure of it, whether I liked it or not.

But making friends meant getting to know people, and getting to know people meant answering questions. And everyone who had seen me for the last few months always asked the same thing.

"How do you manage to sit here and read books all day?"

What am I supposed to say? I thought. *That I'm an ex–psychiatric patient who got wrapped up in a huge insurance scam?*

"I work from home," I said.

But it was a lie. I didn't work. Not yet.

The day before my thirtieth birthday, I woke late to find Nathan sitting in front of the TV. He was watching the news and speaking to someone on the phone.

"Hang on, Mom," he said. "Banning's up. He hasn't seen it yet."

"Seen what?" I asked.

He covered the phone. "Just sit down. You'll see."

I kept my eyes fixed on the television while I sat at my computer. There was a skyscraper with a gaping black hole in it. Tendrils of dark gray smoke curled up its sides, and a huge white antenna pointed into the sky, grim and defiant. The video cut to a plane flying low over New York City. I pictured my dad wearing his uniform, sitting in the cockpit as the plane slammed into the side of the building. A wave of fear swept through me. Nathan was still talking to his mom, but I couldn't hear him. I was a thousand miles away.

"What airline was it?" I asked.

"American," Nathan said, his voice far away.

I think Dad flies for Delta now.

The television stayed on all day. Nathan and I never left the apartment. He went to bed that night, but I lay next to Tundra and stared at the ceiling, thinking about my dad and all the times we had flown together, back when he would put his hat on my head and walk me down the aisle to my seat. I thought about calling him, but I was too afraid he would hang up on me, so I closed my eyes and tried to sleep, only to hear people screaming on the streets of New York City, just like Sonia in the hospital.

I drove to Jennifer's grave two days later. I stopped and bought a dozen white roses like I always did. The front of the store was filled with newspapers featuring photos of the twin towers. The cashier was reading one of them and she looked up at me and then glanced at my flowers and smiled. She didn't say a word. Even the hour-long drive to the cemetery felt different. The weather was beautiful and the streets were empty. The world seemed quieter now.

"I feel helpless," I told Jennifer, lying in the grass next to her grave. "I want to do something, but what can *I* do? A lot of people are talking about joining the military." I rolled onto my back and gazed at the sky. "My dad was in the navy, but I don't know why he joined. He never talked to me about it."

I went home that afternoon and dug through my closet, looking for Dad's needlepoint, which I had hidden behind a pile of boxes. I must have sat on my bed for half an hour, staring at that portrait of me with my reluctant smile and seventies bowl cut, wondering what I would say to my dad if I called him. Then I realized I didn't know anything about him. He had never seen me drive a car or shave or hold a girl's hand. He didn't even know about Jennifer. But I still remembered his phone number, even though I hadn't called him in fifteen years.

I waited for Nathan to go to work the next day, then sat on the floor with Tundra and my cordless phone. For months I had talked to strangers at Starbucks and the girls across the hallway, but my dad didn't even seem real anymore. He was a memory now, a ghost. But the moment he answered the phone, I knew it was him. His voice hadn't changed, although he sounded older now.

"Hey, Dad," I said. "It's Banning."

I don't know why, but I expected him to hang up. Instead his voice rose an octave.

"Banning!" he said. "Hi, son! How are you?"

Holy shit. He still remembers me.

"I just got in from feeding the horses," he said. "I'm sure glad I didn't miss your call. Where are you living now?"

"I live in Fort Worth." I stood and started pacing. "You guys still in the house?"

"Yep. Linda's out working in the barn right now. She'd love to talk to you. We were just talking about you the other day. Your birthday was just last week, wasn't it?"

"Yeah. Just turned thirty."

"Well, happy belated birthday," he said. "You're catching up to your old man." He chuckled and then fell quiet for a moment. "I hope you don't mind my asking, but what ever happened with the lawsuit?"

"We settled out of court a long time ago," I said. "I put most of my money in an annuity."

Dad didn't say anything, so I mentioned I had gotten the needlepoint he had sent me.

"I was hoping you got it," he said. "I always wanted you to have it."

There was a long pause. I wondered if he was as nervous as I was.

"I was calling because of what happened in New York," I said.

Dad groaned. I'd never heard him sound so sad. "It's terrible, all those people. It's just heartbreaking."

"A lot of people are talking about going into the military. It made me wonder why you joined the navy."

There was another pause, but it wasn't awkward this time. I pictured my dad, the dad I remembered, leaning back in his chair and smiling.

"I was twenty-two," he said. "I was almost done with college, but I didn't know what I wanted to do with my life, so I took a break and wound up getting a job on a sailboat. The *Flying Cloud*. I'd never sailed before, but I'd always loved the water. We sailed from southern California to Tahiti. It took twenty-nine days. Anyway, two of the guys on the boat were pilots. They'd spend all day talking about flying. Well, the Vietnam War was going on and a lot of my friends were getting drafted, and I was so close to finishing college that I figured I could get my degree and become a pilot. So when we landed in Tahiti, I flew home and finished my last semester and then signed up for the navy."

Dad spoke as if no time had passed, meandering from one story to the next, about his years in college and the military and friends he once knew. I shared some memories of our going hiking and sailing together, but the moment I finished he grew quiet and started talking about himself again. I could tell he felt guilty, and for some reason that made me feel better. But more than that, I wanted to know if he still cared. And now, after not speaking to each other for fifteen years, there was something about the way he avoided reminiscing about my childhood that hinted at all the love and regret he wasn't willing to share with me. At least not yet.

———

With the house behind me and a regular routine, I thought I had finally found my place in the world. I would wake up every day and eat breakfast and then ride my bike to Starbucks and read until people began getting off work. Sometimes I would stay and talk to some of my friends. Then I'd pick up dinner on the way home and watch the news while I ate. Aside from being a thirty-year-old retiree, my life seemed pretty normal.

But there were other times, days when I would sit outside and listen to the rain or watch the trees sway in the wind, and I would think back to all the times I had gone hiking with my dad, when we used to wander around the land near our house, through the hills and valleys dotted with oak trees and dry creek beds. I hadn't thought about those places since I was in the hospital, back when I used to rock my chair and stare out the window and imagine what it would be like to be free again. Yet here I was—free again—reading books and drinking coffee, as if there were nothing more to do with my life than waste my days away.

20

Countless Pine Trees

More than five years passed after I talked to my dad after 9/11. I had hoped my reaching out to him would bring us together, but he never called me back. In fact, if he hadn't told me about his days in the navy and sailing to Tahiti, I probably would have given up on him. But those stories lived on in my memory, like the image of my friend Jonathan standing by a river in Yosemite. I wanted to do things like that someday, something more beautiful than just living from day to day.

I made small changes at first. I began going on dates and talking about my past. I bought a bike and rode twenty miles every day. Then, after months of learning how to live a normal life, I finally found the courage to leave Fort Worth. I had been dating a girl for a few months when she asked me to move to Austin with her. Two years passed before our relationship began to slowly deteriorate, and she moved out and my life fell apart again. I spent months trying to recover until I finally pulled my Bronco into the garage and closed the door behind me with the engine still running. But instead of waiting to fall unconscious and die in my garage, I yanked the keys out of the ignition and reminded myself of the promise I had made years before.

I can't let the doctors win.

The next morning I went to speak to the woman who managed my apartment complex. She was standing outside the office when I found her.

"I need to move," I said. "If I don't, you're going to find me dead in the apartment."

She stared at me for a long time, trying to figure out if I was joking. Her smile faded. "You're serious, aren't you?"

I nodded.

"Come inside. We'll do the paperwork now," she said. "I won't even charge you for breaking your lease. I'll have someone in your apartment next month."

I gave away or sold most of what I owned before moving back to Dallas later that month in a U-Haul filled with Jennifer's four-poster bed, boxes full of CDs and books, and a small cedar chest that contained Tundra's ashes. She had started having seizures when she was thirteen, and after a dozen trips to the vet and medication that never seemed to help, I finally had to put her to sleep. I sat on the floor of the vet's office and held her in my arms and wept for an hour. She had always been there for me, and I had never forgiven myself for getting angry at her years before. But with her passing, I also knew I had lost one more excuse to stay in Texas. I left Austin and returned to Dallas and rented a small apartment, and I began searching for a place to live—somewhere other than Texas, somewhere I could build a life made of something other than memories.

It was December, just a few weeks before Robert's birthday, when I called him from Dallas. I hadn't seen him since I'd left Austin months before. He had moved in with his partner, Barry. When I lived in Austin, they would invite me over for dinner every weekend. I liked Barry. He was kind and soft-spoken and he loved and respected Robert. They had been together for a few years when Robert contracted a staph infection during a routine visit to the doctor. Then, after developing cellulitis in his legs, he wound up in the hospital. Every time I went to visit him, Barry would be sitting by his side, with his well-kept white hair and bright blue eyes. Robert reassured me everything was fine, and that was enough for me. I still trusted him more than anyone else, even though he kept urging me to give my dad another chance.

The phone rang for about twenty seconds before Barry finally answered. He said Robert was taking a nap, but it was time to get him up. He set down the phone and I could hear them speaking in the background. Robert picked up a moment later. His voice was quiet and tired.

"Hey, Ban. How's life in Dallas?"

"Oh, it's great," I joked. "I just love it here."

He laughed. "It's only temporary. You'll find a place to settle down."

"Not here. I can't fucking stand it here. It feels like a black hole."

"That's not Dallas's fault."

"I know," I said. "I just have so many bad memories here. I can't drive a block without seeing something that reminds me of Jennifer or the hospital."

"Have you ever thought about moving back to California?"

I was hurt. I thought Robert always wanted me nearby.

"I guess," I said. "My friend Jonathan lives there. Nathan moved back there too."

"You could see your dad, also. You should give him a call."

I hated when Robert mentioned my dad. It irritated me. He knew I didn't like talking about him.

"He's the one who dropped me off at the airport," I said. "Why should I keep calling him when he's the one who got rid of me?"

Robert paused for a moment. "Don't you think there might be more to the story than him just getting rid of you? After all, he sent you the needlepoint."

"Maybe, but why doesn't he ever call me? I'm the one who had to call him after 9/11."

"Ban, have you ever considered he might be afraid? I'm not saying you don't have every right to be upset and never talk to him again. You do. But then you'll never talk to him again." He paused again to make sure I'd heard him. "You've always told me how similar you two are. I bet you're both so afraid of losing one another that you don't want to reach out and take a chance."

Since the day I had met Robert in his office eighteen years before, he had always done the same thing. He would plant an idea in my mind and then leave it to grow, like a weed in the crack of a sidewalk. I knew he had a point, but I was tired of reaching out to someone who had dropped me off at the airport and then given me a dollar to call my mom. I had a dad who loved me now. I didn't need another one, especially when he didn't even care enough to call me.

Robert always loved to say "There's two sides to fall off a horse." It was one of a handful of phrases he kept ready for just the right moment.

He once added that I had found a third side to fall off a horse, that I could go to extremes most people couldn't tolerate. I could stare at a wall for months. I could be alone for years. He also said I could endure things that would slowly ruin my life. "You wouldn't have been able to survive the hospital forever," he once told me. "But you survived long enough, and that's what mattered."

Yes, I'd been able survive the hospital, but that skill was ruining my life now. I'd grown so accustomed to tolerating pain that I couldn't identify when something was truly harming me, until the pain grew so intolerable that I wound up on my bed with a gun in my mouth. That first brush with suicide was the first time I knew something was wrong, so I chose to sell the house instead of killing myself. But once I recovered from saying goodbye to Jennifer and all the memories we never made, I settled into a routine that required as little risk as possible, because it was easier to be unhappy than it was to change.

My breakdown in Austin was the second time I almost killed myself, and I walked away from it feeling even more convinced that I needed to change my life. Dating people and riding my bike to Starbucks wasn't enough to numb the pain anymore. I felt like a spacecraft slowly breaking up in an ever-thickening atmosphere. I was thirty-nine years old. I was single. I didn't have a job or a purpose. I had wasted years of my life doing the same inconsequential things to avoid feeling even the slightest amount of pain. But for the first time, after leaving Austin and moving back to Dallas, instead of settling into a familiar routine, my desire to build a new life was stronger than my fear.

I knew I had the courage to move back to California now. I just needed to find a place that felt like home.

———

Robert's birthday passed and January arrived. Late one night, I crawled into bed and turned on the television. Since moving back to Dallas, I had read over a dozen books and watched twice as many documentaries, but I still had no idea what I wanted to do with my life. I sat up in bed and scrolled through a queue crowded with more movies than I could ever watch. I had passed most of them several times and never given them a second thought. But that night, as I passed Ken Burns's documentary about the national parks, I doubled back and pressed play.

The first episode opened with a montage of beautiful locations, like the steaming pools of Yellowstone and the volcanic shorelines of Hawaii. Then, as the narrator began telling the story of a man named Lafayette Bunnell, I scrambled to find the remote among the sheets and then paused the film on a single frame, my heart pounding in my throat.

Countless pine trees dusted with snow lined a deep U-shaped valley. Towering granite walls and spires surrounded the gorge, so large the giant evergreens looked tiny in comparison. To the right and in the distance, a frail and nearly frozen waterfall drifted to the valley floor. Its windblown mist seemed to take minutes to reach the ground.

I stared at the image as a single thought formed itself in my mind.

I'm going to make that place my home.

That place was Yosemite Valley. And even though I had never been there, some part of me sensed that happiness had been left there for me to find.

I rewatched the scene a dozen times before finishing the episode and going to sleep. Before I got out of bed the next morning, I knew what I would be doing that day. I made a pot of coffee and sat down with my laptop and typed two words into the search bar: backpacking Yosemite.

On the first page was a familiar name. REI. The co-op ran retail stores that specialized in outdoor gear. I'd recently started wandering their aisles, gazing at stoves and backpacks and daydreaming of days spent far away from Dallas. The company offered guided trips as well, but I didn't want a guided trip. I wanted to *guide* trips. I wanted a purpose, not a vacation.

I haven't worn a backpack since I was ten years old, I reminded myself. *And I've never even been to Yosemite.*

I clicked on one of the links and scrolled through pictures of granite peaks and smiling clients. The trips were divided into locations within the park: Yosemite Falls, Half Dome, and the high country. One emotional review after the next recounted trips that changed people's lives. Several of them mentioned a guide named Sandy.

I opened another browser and typed "Sandy REI backpacking Yosemite." Halfway down the list was a Facebook page for a woman named Sandy Carpenter. Her bio included references to Yosemite and a guiding company called Valley Adventures, along with dozens of photographs of alpine lakes and sunsets.

I went downstairs and made lunch and thought about what I would say to Sandy. When I sat at my laptop an hour later, I sent her a message and introduced myself, explaining that I wanted to learn how to backpack, and that while I'd be happy to book one of her trips, I preferred to do something more permanent with my life. Somewhere toward the end of the message, I mentioned I'd be willing to share my story if she didn't mind reading a longer email.

Minutes later, as I read and reread the message I had sent, she responded.

Fire away! As long as you're doing the typing, I'll read it. Any life worth living has a grand story behind it. Mine does as well.

I poured every emotional detail of my life into a message so long that it exceeded Facebook's maximum word count, so I sent it in two parts. I shared memories of the hospital and the first time I went outside. I explained the lawsuit, the settlement, and that I would happily work for free. I simply wanted to live my life outdoors and help others do the same.

An hour later Sandy replied again.

Your story was moving to say the least, but a gal has to be careful on the internet. This little business has gone bonkers the last few years and I'm looking for guides with a passion for the wilderness and sharing it with others. I met some of my guides as clients on trips, folks who didn't really know how to backpack. Backpacking I can teach. The passion has to be there, as well as the availability. You seem to have both.

Before signing off, she said if I was ever in the Bay Area that we should meet for lunch. I jumped to my feet and danced in place, then thought of my dad. *This is my chance to call him again,* I thought. But the idea seemed stupid when I considered all the times he had never reached out to me. Then I remembered Robert's advice.

He's probably just as afraid as you are.

I grabbed my phone and dialed Dad's number before I could stop myself. He answered on the first ring. I almost hung up. When I finally managed to say hello, his voice rose an octave, just like it had when I called him after 9/11.

"Banning! How are you, son?"

"I'm good. I'm living in Dallas now," I said.

"I never heard back from you after you called last time. I've been wondering how you're doing."

I almost asked why he never called me, but I was too afraid to ask. I didn't want him to push me away. I told him about Sandy and Yosemite.

"Holy cow, son. A backpacking guide. What a job that'd be."

"Yeah, I'm pretty excited," I said. "I was gonna fly out for the interview soon and I wanted to see if . . ."

He cut me off. "Why don't you stay here at the house? It'd be great to see you again."

My dad didn't seem to realize that he hadn't gone out of his way to contact me in over twenty years. I wanted to see him, but his invitation left me with more questions than answers.

If he's so happy to see me, then why doesn't he ever call?

Sandy had recommended a few dates when she'd be available, so I booked my flight while Dad and I finished talking. He stopped me again when I offered to rent a car.

"Don't worry about that," he said. "Just take the Airport Express shuttle to the Petaluma Fairgrounds. I'll pick you up there and we'll grab lunch at Pearl's. You can have the Mustang all weekend." He paused for a moment. "Come to think of it, we never made it to Yosemite, did we?"

"Nope. Banff, Anchorage, Kalispell, Anza-Borrego. More places than I can remember. But we never went to Yosemite."

"Wow," he said, before whistling a long, descending note. "Just wait till you see it."

Two weeks later I stepped out of the San Francisco airport and stood in the shade of the terminal. The air was cool and smelled of eucalyptus trees and the ocean. I searched for the Airport Express shuttle and then sat in the front seat and gazed out the windshield as the bus headed north through San Francisco and Marin and into the golden hills of Sonoma.

I had no idea what I would say to my dad when I saw him. I wasn't even sure what he looked like now. I hadn't seen him in over twenty years. He was more foreign to me than a stranger, someone I was supposed to know but didn't. In my mind, he was still a young man in a pilot's uniform, standing on the deck of a carrier somewhere in Vietnam.

The shuttle turned in to the fairgrounds and I looked through the crowd at the bus stop for my dad, but I didn't see him. The driver stopped and then stepped out of the bus and handed everyone their bags while we waited in the sunlight. I scanned the people around me, my stomach twisted in knots. I was about to check my phone to see if Dad had called when I heard his voice.

"Hey, son," he shouted.

I turned to see him standing next to a two-door Jaguar convertible with the top down. He was still tall and thin and his arms were long and sinewy like mine. We looked even more alike than we used to, except he was older and had gray hair. I was probably an inch taller than him now.

He shook his head and laughed. "It's like looking at myself thirty years ago."

"Yeah, I was just thinking the same thing," I said.

He gave me a hug. "It's good to have you here, son."

I couldn't recall the last time I had hugged my dad, if it had been at the hospital or when he dropped me off at the airport and sent me to Texas, but I still remembered his sandpaper whiskers on my face and the smell of his skin.

"How was your flight?" he said, letting me go.

"Not bad for United, but they bounced the landing." It was our old joke.

We walked to the car and Dad tossed my bag in the back seat. It was difficult to talk over the sound of the wind, so we sat in silence while Dad drove. Sometimes he'd turn and look at me and smile, but he never said anything. He'd just shake his head and laugh to himself. Twenty minutes later we drove through Sonoma, past vineyards and barns, until we pulled up in front of a vaguely familiar building.

"I'm gonna to go to the restroom," he said. He pointed at a group of tables. "Grab us a spot outside and order whatever you'd like. Oh, and get me an Arnold Palmer, will you, please?"

I was sitting down when a waiter arrived. I ordered Dad's drink and then scanned one of the menus and asked for a patty melt with onion rings instead of fries. Dad returned a moment later, so I went to the restroom while he chatted with the waiter. He had already ordered when I returned.

"So, a backpacking guide in Yosemite, huh?" he said.

"I hope so. We'll find out. I'm meeting Sandy tomorrow."

"Sounds like a great way to spend the summer. Does it pay well?"

"I don't think so," I said. "But it doesn't matter to me. I'd do it for free."

Dad fidgeted with his drink. "I don't mean to pry, but . . . what ever happened with the lawsuit? I never learned much other than what I saw in the news."

He had asked the same question when I called him after 9/11, but he didn't seem to remember, so I told him about the annuity and the bankruptcy years later. He had never found out about the doctors suing me.

He sat there and listened and shook his head in disbelief. The few times I mentioned any details about the hospital, about sitting chair or listening to Sonia, he would wince in pain like I had stuck a knife in his ribs. We were still talking when our waiter arrived holding a tray of food. Dad pulled his chair up to the table as if the conversation were over. The waiter glanced at our order written on a ticket and looked at us, then looked at the ticket again.

"Two patty melts, both with onion rings instead of fries. Did we get that wrong?"

Dad and I burst into laughter. We had ordered the same thing. The waiter chuckled and then set down our orders and walked away. When we finished our meal, I offered to pay but Dad refused. He shoved his card into the little black binder that held our ticket and handed it to the waiter, then started fidgeting with his drink again, even though it was nothing but a bunch of ice cubes now.

"You know, son, if I'd known what was happening in that place, I never would've left you there. They told me you were depressed and suicidal. I didn't know what else to do. I thought I was doing the right thing."

"It's not your fault," I said. "Out of all the kids in our case, Robert said only one of us got pulled out of there by our parents."

Dad sat back in his chair and looked across the street.

"What was your doctor's name again?" he said.

"Dr. Fisher."

"Fisher. That's right," he said, still looking away. "I remember telling her, 'As a pilot, passengers get on my plane and put their lives entirely in my hands. Now I'm forced to do the same thing. You're telling me my son's depressed, and your opinion is all I have. You don't have an X-ray or an MRI to show me what's wrong, so I have no choice but to trust you, the same way my passengers trust me.'"

I told him it wasn't his fault again, but Dad seemed convinced he had done something wrong. Mom felt the same way. Both of my parents had hurt me, but their mistakes seemed trivial compared with the hospital. I'd spent years trying to understand that place, only to realize there was nothing to understand. No one could possibly believe that spending weeks or months facing a wall or tied to a bed was anything other than abuse. And while I would always wonder what my life would have been like if things had been different, it hurt to see my dad take his first steps into that absurd abyss.

We finished lunch and then drove to the house. Dad showed me around. When I asked if anyone else was home, he said Linda and Emily had gone to the grocery store, and Henry had joined the military years before and moved away. We were sitting on the deck behind the barn when a car pulled into the driveway.

"Sounds like the girls are here," he said.

I followed Dad downstairs and through the stables, my stomach in knots again. I had never met Emily, and the last time I recalled seeing Linda was in the hospital. Even from a distance they looked similar, with their blond hair and blue eyes and sunny personalities. Emily ran up the driveway and threw her arms around me, squeezing me as if to make up for all our years apart. I loved her for doing that. Linda was right behind her. She waited for Emily to let go of me and then held me for a long time. I almost pulled away, but I also hoped that she felt differently about me now, that she wanted me in her life, although I didn't know what to believe. More than twenty years had passed since I'd seen

Linda. Hugging me wasn't going to change that. I didn't hate her, but being related by blood or marriage didn't matter to me anymore, not after meeting Robert and Julie and the kids. Family meant something new to me now. And I was sure that no matter what Dad or Linda said, I could never see them the same way again.

21

The Valley

I had just finished working in the barn the next day when a Toyota SUV pulled into the driveway and parked in front of the house. The driver's-side door swung open and two dirty hiking boots appeared, followed by a pair of legs nearly as long as I was tall. On the other end of them was Sandy Carpenter, all six feet of her, grinning as she walked toward me in a T-shirt and what appeared to be a homemade skirt with a pocket stitched to the front. On the back of her SUV was a bumper sticker that read "Chaos, Panic, and Disorder. My Work Here Is Done."

Sandy and I had already exchanged several emails and spoken on the phone. And while I was confident we would get along, I still wasn't sure if she would hire me. I was also afraid of what she might say to my dad. Sandy was fiery and outspoken and had two college-aged kids. To her, the idea of leaving her children in an institution seemed unfathomable. So when I invited her to the house, I asked her not to say anything about my parents or the hospital.

"I'll do my best," she said over the phone, "but I can't promise anything. My mouth has a mind of its own sometimes."

We had barely finished shaking hands when Dad came strolling out of the house. He offered to give Sandy a tour of the ranch, so I trailed behind them while she talked about going to college and meeting her husband and guiding in Yosemite. When Dad mentioned he swam in college, Sandy lit up like a Christmas tree. "I swam in high school," she said. Soon they stopped in the shade of the barn and leaned on the gate of the horse pasture while I pretended to clean one of the stalls and eavesdropped. One of the farm cats interrupted their conversation, and when Sandy reached down to pet him, she noticed me standing nearby.

"Ready to head down to the plaza for lunch?" she asked. "I'm happy to drive."

"Yeah, I figured we'd go to the Cheese Factory for a sandwich or something, if that sounds okay?"

She nodded and then turned on her heel and strode back to her SUV. When I sat and buckled my seat belt, I looked over to see her staring out the windshield, lost in thought.

"It's hard to believe someone who'd leave their kid at the airport could be so nice," she said finally.

"I don't know. After our lunch yesterday, I'm starting to think I've been wrong about my dad for a long time."

She turned and looked at me. "Parents don't leave their kids at the airport. Not good parents, anyway."

Sandy cranked the ignition and headed downhill into town. She asked about my childhood and the days I had spent outside with my dad. But no matter what I said about all the good things he had done, she would just clench her jaw and stare out the windshield. I understood why people disliked my parents. They both had made terrible mistakes, but I still felt the need to defend them, probably because I was still trying to understand where my resentment ended and my love began.

Sandy circled the plaza before we managed to find a parking spot.

"I think I'm gonna grab a table outside," I said. "I don't really like sitting inside. It's too noisy."

Sandy grinned. "You sound like a backpacker."

She disappeared inside the restaurant while I stood in line at the grill. After getting my food, I carried my plate to the end of the patio and found a table away from the others. Sandy stepped outside a few minutes later and set her sandwich on the table and pulled up a chair.

"So how long did you live here in Sonoma?" she asked.

"Only a year or so. Dad and Linda got married down there at the mission right before we moved here." I tipped my head at a nearby white adobe chapel. "I was the ring bearer. Dad had a running bet on how many times I'd drop the ring, since I could never sit still. Three times. He won."

Sandy smiled and nodded politely, the way people do when they're thinking something they don't want to share. She turned to her sandwich.

"So how did you get into backpacking?" I asked.

Sandy's eyes lit up and she burst into a grin. She hid her mouth behind her napkin.

"It started with this guy named Ken Hart," she said, still chewing. "He was in my English class in high school. Our teacher gave us an assignment to demonstrate something we liked, and Ken showed up with a backpack. I still remember watching him walk to the front of the classroom and drop it on the teacher's desk and say, 'This is a backpack, and this is what I do.' I was amazed. He was showing us some of his gear when someone shouted, 'Where do you go?'" Sandy paused and shook her head and laughed. "'Anywhere I want,' he told us. I was sold. The minute he said it I remember thinking, *This is what I'm meant to do.* Until that day, my mother had controlled every aspect of my life. Everything I did was scheduled and had to be perfect. I didn't know the freedom Ken was talking about was even possible."

Sandy leaned back in her chair and turned to watch some kids playing in the park across the street. She sat there for a while, smiling as if they reminded her of something. She was still watching them when she spoke again.

"My mother used to spend every Thanksgiving cooking all day and fussing over everything. She'd set the table and double-check each piece of silverware and china and crystal. Then, with the turkey and all the food sitting there like the cover of *Better* fucking *Homes & Gardens*, she'd take a picture of the table with no one sitting at it. She did it every year. No people. No family. No smiles. The photo was better without us."

I don't remember what I had imagined it would be like to meet Sandy, but it didn't involve a heart-to-heart about our dysfunctional parents or their holiday traditions. We had spent less than an hour on the phone and only exchanged a handful of emails, yet anyone sitting nearby would have thought we were old friends.

"Sorry about that," she said, wiping her eyes with her napkin. "You're probably wondering why you flew out here to play therapist to some old lady."

"No, it's okay. I understand."

"I know you do," she said. "That's probably why I'm sitting here blubbering. Honestly, sometimes I wonder why anyone would work for me. I'll never understand how I managed to bring together such an amazing group of guides. I could've just hired a bunch of jocks to haul around packs for people, but that's not how I run my business. A good guide isn't a pack mule. We're teachers. And we don't just teach people how to navigate in the mountains. We teach people how to take care of themselves. We're out there showing them how to do it, not doing it for them. I want to give folks permission to cry and be vulnerable, things I was never allowed to do."

Before I'd boarded the plane to meet Sandy and see my dad, I'd convinced myself the entire trip would be a failure. Dad wouldn't pick me up at the bus stop and Sandy wouldn't hire me. After all, only strong, capable people with years of experience worked as backpacking guides in Yosemite National Park. It wasn't a job for an ex–psychiatric patient. I'd have to help people and talk to them. But I was so desperate to build a new life and spend time outdoors that I didn't care about being alone anymore. And after meeting Sandy and listening to her story, I began to realize there were other people who were just as wounded as me.

She pushed her plate out of the way and then dug through her purse and pulled out a small map of Yosemite. She set it on the table in front of me and tapped it like a deck of cards.

"Remember in your email when you said you feel like you don't have a real family? Well, once you start guiding, you're going to realize you get to have a new family every week."

I flew back to Texas to wait out the five months before my first season as a guide. Dad and Linda agreed to let me have the room above the barn for the summer, and because I'd need my car to commute to and from Yosemite, I planned on driving to California in May and then returning home in September. But I didn't have a home in Texas. All I had was an apartment, a small group of friends, and a girl I'd started dating a few months before. That's not to say they weren't important to me. They were. But somewhere in the back of my mind I'd always known I'd return to California. And not just for the season but forever.

I did have two friends who lived in California, though. Jonathan had settled in Monterey, and Nathan had moved to Los Angeles and graduated from film school. But they had lives now. We weren't going to live together and play games all day or hang out all the time. I'd have to build a new life in California, away from all the people and places I'd known for so long. I couldn't help but feel like a coward. I'd just gotten a job as a backpacking guide in Yosemite National Park, and all I could think about was how terrified I was to finally leave the one place I'd never wanted to live.

It wasn't lost on me that I'd been afraid to leave the hospital too. My friends and I hated being there. But when the time came for us to go home or to a halfway house, we'd hesitate or panic. Some kids even burst into tears and grabbed the doors as their parents dragged them away. Many of us had come from broken or abusive families, and after years of hardship, anything remotely close to a normal life felt strange. So much of my identity had been built upon suffering that the idea of being happy seemed wrong. Only in my earliest memories could I remember a time when I didn't feel broken. The idea of lasting happiness didn't even make sense to me. Happiness was something temporary that briefly interrupted long stretches of loneliness and pain. Building a new life and being happy not only seemed impossible; it felt like a betrayal of all my friends from the hospital, especially Jennifer.

I called Robert before I left for California. He was living with Barry in Arkansas now, and they were building a house on some land near his mom's place. He was still struggling with his health, but his voice was bright when he answered the phone.

"I'll be leaving Dallas in a few weeks," I said. "But I'm coming back to Texas at the end of the season. Maybe I can come visit soon."

"That'd be nice, Ban. You're always welcome here."

"I don't know what I'm going to do when I get back. I don't even know *why* I'm coming back. I hate this place, but it's all I've got right now."

"One step at a time," he said. "There's a reason you moved back there after you left Austin. You may not love Dallas, but it was your home for a long time. You have friends there. Jennifer's there too. You can't just tear up all those roots and move away in a few weeks. It takes time to say goodbye."

"I guess you're right," I said. "I'm just scared."

"Of course you are, Ban. You're growing."

It was mid-April when I loaded my car full of new backpacking gear and set out for California. By the time I made it to Sonoma, two days and one hotel later, my car was covered in four states' worth of dirt and bugs, and a rock had cracked my windshield.

The morning after I arrived, Dad put me to work. We spent my first week at the house repairing the barn and trimming trees and clearing brush out of the pasture. We'd eat lunch together every day, and at five o'clock we'd sit on the deck and have a cocktail while he worked his way through a dog-eared book of sudoku puzzles. I loved those afternoons. Sometimes I'd sit there quietly and wonder why I'd waited so long to reach out to him. Other times he'd tell me stories about his years in the navy.

"When we first moved to Orange County, I used to buzz our neighborhood when I was out on training flights," he said, laughing. "They started writing about it in the papers. I would have gotten in a lot of trouble if I ever got caught."

"How old was I?" I asked.

"Barely a year old, I think. I doubt you'd remember."

"I still have tons of memories of living there," I said. "I remember when we'd go swimming at night and we could see the fireworks from Disneyland over the fence. Or the time that gopher snake got loose in the house and Mom wouldn't come out of the bedroom."

Dad watched me for a moment and then smiled and turned back to his book. He didn't say a word. He had done the same thing when I called him after 9/11. But now, as we sat there together on the deck behind the barn, something in his smile told me that those memories truly were as precious to him as they were to me, and that he just wasn't ready to talk about them yet. So I sat back in my chair and watched him ponder over that dog-eared book of sudoku puzzles while I built some new memories. Rehashing my childhood didn't seem worth ruining whatever future we had left.

Dad and I had just finished working one afternoon when Sandy called to see if I wanted to join her and a couple of friends for a two-night backpacking trip. Our guiding season was only a few weeks away, and she mentioned we'd be close to Yosemite and might have a chance to stop and see the valley on our way home.

"It's a short hike in and out," she said. "Maybe it'll give you a chance to try out some of your new gear."

The next day I sat in the passenger seat as we wound our way through the Bay Area and into the Central Valley. Sandy pointed out landmarks that lined the route on the way to the park, like the town of Manteca and the almond groves and fruits stands near Escalon and Oakdale. The drive looked nothing like the pictures I'd seen of Yosemite. There were no waterfalls in the distance or granite peaks. Instead, it was flat and hot and smelled like cattle. Three hours later, after we had parked at the trailhead and gotten out of the car, I was convinced Yosemite was still hundreds of miles away. When I mentioned it to Sandy, she grinned and pointed up the hill.

"The park's only about ten minutes away," she said.

I hadn't gone backpacking since I was a child, and I'd bought my gear after reading some blogs about "essential" backpacking equipment. Sandy asked to see my pack, and she unloaded it and started tossing things to the side.

"Nope. Nope. Don't need this either." She held up a new roll of toilet paper. "How much are you gonna shit in two days? Take half this much and pull the cardboard out of the middle. That's useless."

By the time we had finished, my pack weighed half as much, but I felt naked.

"Look," Sandy said, "people don't need half the stuff they think they do. And if I'm wrong, the car's right here. It's a short walk in and out. Three miles, max. If you need something, we'll come back and get it."

I glanced at my pack again. Inside it was everything I needed to survive. Clothes. Food. A sleeping bag. A handful of other things. I lifted the pack and shook it. It didn't weigh much. I remember thinking I had spent most of my life learning how to survive, only to realize that I'd never needed very much. And that all the things I'd thought were necessary, like my years of being alone, had actually been weighing me down.

A car pulled up and two old men got out. Sandy waved them over and introduced us. They both had white beards and grinned a lot. They didn't look like the attractive backpackers I'd seen on REI's website. They looked like miners who had gotten lost in the mountains. One was as thin as a board and the other had a potbelly. The latter was Sandy's mentor, she said. I began to wonder what I'd gotten myself into.

We put on our packs and followed a swollen creek lined with pine trees. Sandy's mentor stopped every ten minutes. Sometimes he'd pat my shoulder and point out a butterfly or a flower or teach me something. "Alders like their feet wet," he said once, gesturing to a small tree half submerged in the creek. It turned out he had been a high school biology teacher for more than forty years. He had taken more kids backpacking than he could remember. By the time we reached a small waterfall and set up camp, I'd forgotten half of what he had taught me.

For two days we stayed near our camp and went on short hikes through a nearby valley. Its rim was dotted with snow and pine trees, and I kept staring at them, wondering if I might catch a glimpse of Yosemite in the distance. Sandy and her friends taught me about the plants and trees and geology of the Sierra. At night we'd sit around the campfire and they'd point out stars and constellations.

"The cold air makes the night sky really clear," Sandy said. "It's going to be a hell of a season." She kicked a small patch of snow. "We've gotten almost twice the amount of snow we usually do this year. I can't imagine what's it like in the high country. You chose a hell of a year to become a guide."

"Will you have to cancel trips?" I asked.

She shook her head. "I'll just move 'em to another trailhead. I've already rerouted trips to other parts of the park."

On our last morning we jumped in the creek and lay on the granite and warmed ourselves in the sunlight. I crawled into the shade of the trees and listened to Sandy and her friends share stories about their years of guiding in the mountains and the mistakes they had made and the places they loved. After we dried off, we packed our belongings and walked back to the parking lot, where Sandy and I bade her two friends farewell. Then we threw our stuff in her SUV and headed back to the road we had taken days before. When we stopped at the intersection, she glanced up the hill.

"We have all day," she said. "Let's go see the valley. Maybe we can find a campsite and crash for the night."

We followed a winding, snow-lined road past the entrance of Yosemite and on through miles of forest and mountains. Sandy pointed out campgrounds and sequoia groves and the junction of the Tioga Road. We were driving past a steep ridgeline covered with fallen trees when she lifted a finger from the steering wheel. "There it is," she said. "Half Dome." The peak vanished behind a ridgeline and then reappeared a moment later, its iconic face stained with black streaks and crowned with snow.

"Holy shit. It's huge," I said.

Sandy laughed. "Just wait till you see it up close."

The peak disappeared again and we continued downhill until we came to the floor of the valley. Sandy turned left at a stop sign and then followed the road alongside a river. The water was white and turbulent and the trees that lined its shores swayed in the mist. After crossing a small bridge, she pulled into a turnout beside the road.

"It's tradition to stop at Fern Spring and get a drink," she said.

I opened my door and followed her to a small stream. Overhead, a dense canopy of trees shaded the sun, their leaves dotted with creamy blooms the color of lemon meringue.

"Dogwoods," Sandy said, looking up at them. "They bloom in April. What an amazing month to see the valley for the first time." She knelt at the creek and cupped her hand and took a sip. "Don't worry. It won't make you sick. This was snow just a few minutes ago."

I lowered my hand into the stream. The water was colder than ice. I brought it to my lips and took a sip.

Sandy grinned. "Your first valley baptism."

We walked back to the car and I rolled down my window. I hung my head outside and watched the emerald kaleidoscope of leaves and light overhead. Then, just as we left the woods, Sandy tapped the brakes and said something. It was difficult to hear her over the wind, so I pulled my head inside the car when I saw her pointing at the windshield.

A colossal wall of granite, towering and monstrous, obscured the sky. It loomed thousands of feet over the meadow, its craggy face streaked by millions of years of rain and snow. I stared at the wall, aware of nothing else, wondering if it was something so divine that I should close my eyes. Sandy stopped the car and the engine fell quiet. For minutes I sat there gazing at the peak as tears streamed down my face. It seemed permanent in a way that nothing else ever had, as if it had always existed, unchanged and timeless, and hidden somewhere behind its immense face was something that had always been calling to me, even when I was in the hospital and lying on Jennifer's grave. And now, after years of searching for it, I had finally found it waiting for me, like a sentinel watching over its sacred, beloved home.

"This was here when I was in the hospital," I said, still crying, "when I used to stare out my window. It was here when Jennifer died too. This place has always been here, just waiting."

Sandy smiled and wiped her eyes.

"I know," she said. "That's why I hired you."

22

We're Going to Need More Chips

Days after returning from Yosemite, Sandy invited me to her house for dinner. She and her husband, Ron, lived in the Bay Area, about an hour away from Sonoma. I had only met Ron in passing, so I knew the dinner was sort of an interview.

"Ron's wanted to talk to you ever since you emailed me," Sandy said. "He's curious about your family."

Everyone was curious about my family. I was curious about my family. They made no sense to me. And from what I knew about Ron, they probably wouldn't make sense to him either. Sandy said his father had died when Ron was a child, and when she told him my story, he was angry and confused.

"What am I supposed to tell him?" I asked her.

"The truth," she said.

I arrived at their house the following evening. I could hear Ron playing guitar somewhere in the house. When Sandy answered the door, he strode into the entryway, wearing one of those reluctant smiles that made him look shy and thoughtful. I knew he had a PhD in biochemistry and worked for a biotech firm and played acoustic guitar. He had bright green eyes and a beard dotted with gray hair, and he didn't walk so much as move with purpose, like a man forever walking into the wind.

He waved us into the kitchen and went to work on dinner while Sandy opened a bottle of wine and stayed out of his way. We hadn't made it halfway through our meal when he began asking about my life. But as I retold each part of my story, Ron would interrupt and finish it for me, as if he had memorized everything Sandy had told him. He knew about the airport and the hospital and my mom asking for money. He knew about my dad sending me away. But no matter what I tried to add, he would just shake his head and ask the same questions, his voice quivering in anger. "How could they do that?" "Why do you still talk to them?" "How could they just get rid of you?" He walked to one end of the kitchen and stabbed his finger at the living room sofa. "Sandy and I were sitting right there when she read your first email, when you told her everything. We both cried. They're your parents. How could you just forgive them after everything they've done?"

"I didn't just forgive them," I said. "I don't even know my dad. I think I'm still forgiving him."

Ron shook his head like a child. "No, no, no. I don't buy that. It can't be that easy."

"It's not easy. I know what they did was wrong, but I can't keep hating them. It's fucking exhausting. I spent years hating myself because of everything they did to me. But after a while I figured out that hating my parents wasn't hurting them. It was only hurting me."

I'd never admitted to forgiving my parents, and I didn't often say things without inspecting and approving each phrase. But the moment those words left my mouth, I knew I'd not only forgiven my parents but forgiven everyone. Dr. Fisher. Luther. The orderlies who used to pin down Sonia while she screamed for help. But I also knew that forgiving them wasn't an act of kindness. I'd forgiven them because I was exhausted. I knew I'd never get an apology for anything they had done. Dr. Fisher would never say she was sorry for making me sit alone in my room. My dad would never say he was sorry for leaving me at the airport. My mom would never say she was sorry for demanding money or hitting me. I didn't forgive those people because I loved them. I forgave them because I didn't want the hospital or my parents or their abuse to define me anymore.

Ron looked like he had been struck by lightning. He sat there staring at me, his jade-green eyes wide. Then, after a few seconds, he got up from the table and left the room. I turned and looked at Sandy with my mouth half open.

"Give him some time," she said. "He's still sorting out his own demons."

She didn't say anything else. She just patted me on the shoulder and poured me another glass of wine. Ten minutes later, when Ron walked back into the kitchen, his eyes were red and swollen.

"Someday you'll have to teach me how you forgave your parents," he said. "Because right now, I just don't get it."

When most people think of Yosemite National Park, they picture the same iconic valley I'd visited with Sandy. But that valley occupies less than 1 percent of the park. There are countless other places to explore within Yosemite. And about fifteen miles to the north, in another waterfall-lined valley, there's a place called Hetch Hetchy, and it's where I became a professional guide less than a week after that dinner with Sandy and Ron.

It was tradition for Sandy to lead the first trip of the season, and because it was only my second time in the park, we arrived early that afternoon and unloaded the gear while she explained how to set up a stove and fit a backpack and use a water filter. Two hours later, when the first clients began to arrive, I could barely remember my own name.

"Don't worry," she said, putting one of her long arms around my shoulder. "You're sharp. Just stay near me and watch. You'll have it in no time."

For the rest of the trip, I was Sandy's secret apprentice. I'd smile and introduce myself to clients and then run back to her like a scared child. I mimicked everything she did. She'd volunteer someone and then rummage through their backpack, explaining what they needed and what they didn't. She'd toss aside their flannel pajamas and hardcover books with the same friendly disdain she'd had for my new roll of toilet paper. "Nope. Nope. Don't need this either." Some clients stood there in tears, clutching their iPhones or mascara, and Sandy would talk them down like a hostage negotiator. I made mental notes of everything she said, since unbeknownst to the clients, I knew as little as they did.

The next morning we threw on our packs and hiked into the Hetch Hetchy valley. For three days it rained, sleeted, and snowed. Every morning we ate breakfast around a damp, smoky campfire. Then we'd pack our lunches and leave camp to explore the valley for a few hours, only to come back and eat dinner around the same sad campfire. Shivering clients woke me in the middle of the night. "I'm freezing," they'd whisper through their clenched teeth. I'd get up and make them a hot water bottle over a stove I hardly knew how to use. Then, holding the bottle like a newborn, they'd curl up in their sleeping bag and fall asleep, then I'd pack up the pot and stove and stroll back to my tent, wondering how I could be so happy in the freezing rain at two in the morning.

By the end of the month, I'd spent nearly half my days in Yosemite, working alongside Sandy or one of my fellow guides. Our clients came from all over the world. We began each four-day trip as strangers and finished as friends. We cooked together and laughed together and slept by the same fire. We swam in moonlit lakes and talked about our lives. And although Ron once told me that some people just wanted a vacation, there were always the others who came searching for something that even they didn't understand. Those were the people I most looked forward to meeting, because I didn't really guide them; they guided me. They proposed to each other or celebrated years free of cancer or addiction. Some even scattered the ashes of their loved ones. It was through those people and the wilderness around us that I learned what Sandy meant when she once told me, "The mountains will open your pores." I didn't understand those words at first, but after weeks of witnessing clients opening their hearts to us, I realized why Linda and my dad seemed so distant sometimes. It was because they had never opened their hearts to me. The few times I saw them feel anything like regret or remorse, they quickly changed the subject or cracked a joke. I'd never seen either of them cry. In fact, after four days in the backcountry, I often knew more about my clients than I knew about my own parents. The wilderness required a certain level of hardship. And when everyone had to carry their fair share, and our only concerns were food and water and a comfortable place to rest, the emotional barriers between us seemed unimportant. That intimacy made me feel normal again. Not only because of the conversations that we shared but also because those people became something like a family to me. I was never lonely when I was guiding. I never thought of my parents or the void they had left behind. Every day I lived surrounded by warmth and kindness. Every night I slept among friends. We laughed and cried and supported one another. We were everything a family was supposed to be.

Once, just hours into a trip, a client began to cry as we started across a stream. He looked as big as a mountain, sitting on a log next to his wife, hiding in her arms to conceal his tears. It was only after he spoke to Sandy that he finally got to his feet and crossed the river while he held his wife's hand.

"What's going on?" I asked Sandy when she rejoined our group.

"His brother drowned a few years ago, crossing a river," she said. "He came here to cross one for him."

Before those earliest trips, I'd imagined being a backpacking guide would somehow fix me, that I'd become more like other people by proving that I was capable and strong. I pictured swinging ice axes and pulling folks up snowy peaks, only to have them beam at me in adoration. But after a month of working alongside Sandy and dozens of clients, I learned that people weren't stronger or more capable than me. They were flawed and broken. They were alcoholics or cutters or parents who had alienated their kids. And no matter where they had come from or what they had survived, we all wanted the same thing: a family where we felt like we belonged.

It was a warm July afternoon when I parked in front of the barn next to Dad and Linda's house. I'd left Yosemite that morning and my body was sore from the long drive home. The house looked quiet and all the cars were gone, so I carried my backpack to my room and then swept the barn and cleaned the pasture. I'd promised to help Dad and Linda in exchange for their letting me stay, but I'd been so busy that I hadn't been able to contribute much.

I'd hardly seen them seen since I'd arrived in Sonoma. They were almost always together, and the few times I'd spoken to them alone they acted differently, especially Linda. Away from my dad, her sunny demeanor would fade and she would confide in me about her growing older and looking back on all the mistakes she had made. Once, she even began telling me about the day Dad had driven me to the airport and sent me to Texas.

"I was so young back then," she said. "I didn't know how to be a good mom to you. I was barely thirty years old. I just wanted to be your friend, but then we started arguing. And your dad was always so busy flying, I didn't know what to do. I went to bed in tears almost every night. I felt like a failure."

I was stunned. I sat there in silence, wondering what to say. It was the first time I'd seen Linda act like a human being, someone who wasn't convinced that everything in her life was perfect. Then Dad strolled through the front door and she began to laugh as if she had just told me a joke.

"Hey, honey," she said to him, quickly wiping her eyes. "You boys ready for lunch?"

It was in those brief moments alone with Linda, and in the time I spent on the patio with Dad, that I learned to see them both through different eyes. For most of my life, my dad and stepmom had been nothing but a collection of childhood memories. And like most children, I had always assumed they had a reason for everything they had done. The years of abuse my mom had heaped on me were a living, breathing thing, as real as all the other pain I'd suffered as a teenager and adult. And because of it, I'd learned to see my mom for who she was, a bitter woman who couldn't see beyond her own depression and loneliness. But I didn't know my dad or Linda well, and after living apart for twenty-six years, I wasn't sure if I ever would.

Hours after returning from the park, just as I finished cleaning the pasture, I heard Dad whistle from the barn. I turned to see him standing in the shade, grinning at me.

"Long day, huh?" he said.

"Yeah, I left the park around ten this morning. Then I had to drop off all the gear at Sandy's and help her organize a few things. We have another trip going out tomorrow, but someone else is guiding it, so I have a couple of days off to help around the ranch." A dull twinge of guilt shot through me. "I'm sorry I haven't been around much. I've just been trying to help Sandy as much as I can."

He waved it off. "As long as you're working hard, that's what matters. Anyway, Linda and I just got home and we were hoping you might want to join us for dinner. We were gonna head into town and grab some Mexican food."

I set my rake in one of the empty stalls and followed Dad's backlit silhouette as he ambled through the barn ahead of me. He was old now and moved slowly, hunched forward as if he were carrying something heavy that no one could see. He seemed so frail. I recalled being a child and gazing up at him, the towering pilot in his uniform. It was then that I realized that, just as the hospital had given me a deeper gratitude for my freedom, the years I'd spent apart from my dad had given me a deeper appreciation for him. He wasn't immortal anymore. He wasn't a phantom or ghost. He was a vulnerable old man who had hidden away his memories and regrets, until they had become so heavy that he couldn't seem to carry them any longer.

But alongside my newborn compassion for my father lay a lingering resentment, and reconciling those two emotions seemed impossible. My dad had neglected me for years, and all he had offered me in return was a fragile relationship built on a handful of conversations over dinner and a few moments together on the patio. Some part of me had forgiven him for everything he had done, but another part of me needed something in return, some kind of acknowledgment that he knew what he had done was wrong.

The restaurant was quiet when we arrived. Dad and Linda went straight to the patio and found a table in the shade. It was a warm afternoon. The sun was still high and the patio cover was topped with wavy sheets of green fiberglass that made it look like we were sitting underwater. By the time our food arrived, we'd each finished half a margarita.

"So what's it like being a backpacking guide?" Linda asked.

"It's not what I imagined," I said. "I thought we'd be wandering through the mountains and climbing peaks, but it's more about listening to people. When you spend four days with a bunch of strangers without phones or TVs or showers, everything changes. You get to know people pretty quickly. Each group kind of feels like its own little family."

Linda grinned and shook her head. "I don't think I could go without a shower for that long. I'd go crazy."

"Every trip has a few people who just suffer through it," I said. "But I don't think I'll ever get tired of guiding. It's what I'm meant to do. I never thought I'd figure out what I was supposed to do with my life when I was almost forty."

"That's how I felt when I met Linda," Dad said, reaching for our basket of chips.

He'd said it without even thinking about it, as if they were the truest words to ever leave his mouth. Linda broke into a smile and gave him a peck on the cheek.

"I bet your father never told you how we met," she said.

Dad rolled his eyes.

"He was sitting in the front row of the plane. I'd only been a flight attendant for a few years and I had a horrible argument with my ex that morning. I could barely keep it together. I remember crying during the preflight check. Well, your dad sees me and says, 'Want to get married for twenty-four hours?' I almost slapped him. I stood there staring at him for a few seconds. 'I've been married to one of you assholes before,' I told him, 'and my life is still miserable.'"

Dad put his arm around Linda's shoulder. "She stormed off in tears. I felt terrible. Your mom and I had only been separated for a few months back then. I had a trip the next day, so I swapped flights with a friend so I could see Linda again and apologize. I still loved your mom, Banning, but we never had that kind of relationship. Everything with Linda's always been easy. The next time we met, I knew we'd get married."

"That was a hard time for me. It was for both of us," Linda said. "But we held each other together. Then I met you and your sister Adrienne. I wasn't even thirty years old. God, I was so young. I had no idea what I was doing."

For a moment I considered asking one of the million questions that had been floating around in my mind since the day they had sent me away, but I didn't want to interrupt her. It was almost as if she didn't know she was speaking. Maybe it was the half margarita or the few stories she had already shared with me. But whatever the reason, it was the first time I felt like she wasn't my stepmom. She was just a person who had made mistakes, like the dozens of clients I'd talked to over the summer.

Dad pulled the last few chips out of the basket. He didn't say anything. Linda sat next to him, staring at her margarita.

"Why did you guys send me away?" I asked.

Dad flinched. It was the same expression he'd made when I first mentioned the hospital, like I'd stabbed him. Linda looked at him as if she needed permission to say something.

"We never wanted to tell you," she said. "We were both so afraid."

I leaned forward in my seat. "Tell me what?"

"We never wanted to sound like we were trying to manipulate you or change your mind," she said. "You were only a boy. I never wanted to turn you against your mom."

She looked at dad again. He was staring at the table.

"Your mom used to send me the ugliest letters," Linda continued. "She'd say your dad was still in love with her and that you and Adrienne hated me. I almost didn't marry your dad because of her. It went on for years. It didn't stop until we finally sent you to live in Texas."

"But she didn't want me either," I said. "She tried to send me back to live with you guys."

Dad began fidgeting with his margarita. "She had full custody, son. We had to follow the settlement agreement. We didn't have a choice. While you were in the hospital, we even offered to take you out, but your mom refused."

I froze. A huge pillar of rage came rushing out of me. I almost started screaming at him. I wanted to shove everything off the table, but the expression on Dad's face stopped me. He looked gutted. I didn't know whether to shout at him or cry. I knew he and Linda had made mistakes, and that what they had done was wrong, but it was hard to feel sympathy for them that day. I also knew I'd just gotten the closest thing to an apology I'd ever receive, and that someday I'd be grateful, but not today.

Linda wiped her eyes with a napkin and put her arm around Dad's shoulder. He turned to look at her as if he'd forgotten she was there. Then he let go of his margarita and reached for the basket in the center of the table.

"We're going to need more chips," he said.

23

The Trainwreck Trip

By early September I had guided eleven trips, each of them four days long. Together they covered every itinerary that Sandy had ever created. I had also spent eleven days off-trail with her and Ron and their friends, backpacking across some of the highest portions of the eastern Sierra. The one thing I hadn't done, however, was lead a group, until Sandy called me the week before my birthday and told me she had mistakenly scheduled one of our trips for the wrong date.

"The clients already booked their flights," she said. "They'll be waiting for us in the valley this Friday."

"For what trip?"

She groaned. "Half Dome."

Half Dome was one of the most popular destinations in the park, and all the permits for it had been reserved six months in advance. Trying to get new permits would have been like shopping for tickets to a sold-out concert the night before the show.

"I can't believe this," she said. "What a fucking trainwreck. Every permit for every trailhead near Half Dome is booked full. So I called in a favor, and without going into the details, I got the permits to run it, but it's not our normal itinerary. Do you have a map handy?"

Sandy spent the next hour explaining the trip, along with the trails I'd be using and the landmarks I'd see along the way. The more she told me, the more nervous I became. The forecast was bad. The trip was full. The route was longer than usual and less scenic. If there was any good news, she hadn't shared it with me yet.

"Who's guiding it with me?" I asked.

"Gregor."

He was one of Sandy's best guides. Experienced, quiet, and dependable. He'd guided for her for years.

"Then why isn't he leading?" I asked.

"He's led trips before and doesn't like it. Most of you guides lead together anyway." She lowered her voice. "Don't worry, Banning. You can do this. You're ready."

I almost asked her to take my place, but Sandy disliked Half Dome trips more than any of us did. The route was our most physically demanding and the only one with a single goal: stand on top of Half Dome. When conditions prevented us from making the summit, clients often left disappointed or angry. It could also be dangerous. The route to the summit required using a pair of cables to ascend the last four hundred feet, and a fall would be fatal.

The day before the trip, Sandy emailed me the forecast and client information. The forecast had deteriorated and several of the clients had concerns about whether we would be able to make the summit. When I arrived at Sandy's house the next day to pick up the gear, she handed me a map and a folder of detailed instructions entitled "Trainwreck Half Dome Trip."

"What a fucking birthday present," I grumbled.

"It's your birthday?"

"I'm turning forty on the last day of the trip."

"If I'd known, I wouldn't have asked you," she said.

"Does that mean you'll guide it for me?"

She clapped me on the back. "You'll do fine. You have plenty of experience now. Stop worrying."

Nearly all of Sandy's other guides had full-time jobs. They sacrificed weekends or vacation time to work for her. Meanwhile, I'd spent half my summer in the park, backpacking with clients while the other guides were stuck at work.

Gregor pulled up to the house while Sandy and I were loading the gear into my car. He waved hello and started helping us without saying a word. It was typical Gregor, mellow and easygoing. Just being near him made me feel better. By the time we arrived in Yosemite and found our campsite, I'd forgotten all about Sandy's "Trainwreck" paperwork.

For years Sandy had run her trips using the same formula. Most of the clients didn't know one another, and she had taught us that our first thirty seconds together could make or break the trip, so we always set out appetizers and wine and put on our best smiles. Then we'd sit with the clients and talk about why they wanted to backpack and why they had chosen Yosemite.

Gregor and I had just finished setting out the wine and snacks when the clients began to arrive, so we alternated between checking everyone's gear and introducing ourselves. After months of working for Sandy, I'd learned that a good backpacking guide did a lot more than just lead a group. We were counselors and massage therapists and bartenders and chefs. We patched blisters in the rain and made margaritas using snow. Some clients arrived thinking we'd carry their gear for them, and for the rest of the trip they'd complain about their feet or backpack while we cheered them on. Some people even broke down in tears. Those folks were always my favorites. I loved most everyone, but the look of accomplishment on someone's face after struggling through four days of doubt and suffering never got old for me.

We finished the pack checks and discovered that a few people had forgotten some items, so we agreed to stop by the store before we took the bus to our trailhead in the morning. One of the clients, an older woman with snowy white hair and a sky-blue rain jacket, overheard us. When Gregor and I rejoined our group at the picnic table, she spoke from the far end.

"Why are we taking a bus?" she asked. "I thought we were going over Cloud's Rest."

Cloud's Rest was another popular destination. The narrow granite ridgeline stood a thousand feet taller than Half Dome, and the view from the top was one of the best in the park. But since Sandy had redesigned the trip using different permits, we wouldn't be following the normal itinerary that had been advertised on the REI website.

"We had a problem with the permits," I said. "So we'll be starting from a different trailhead. But we'll see it from Half Dome."

The woman stood up and glared at me. "Then we could make it a day hike."

Another woman, clearly her friend, jumped to her feet and began to calm her down.

"We wouldn't have enough time to make it to our next camp if we took a day hike," I said. "I'm sorry."

The woman narrowed her eyes. She leaned over the far end of the picnic table and pointed at me. I could feel her finger in my chest from five feet away.

"I specifically booked this trip to go over Cloud's Rest!" she shouted. "I've already been up Half Dome! Three fucking times!"

Her friend grimaced and then smiled at me if she had sat on something painful.

"I really am sorry," I said. "But sometimes we have to change our plans, especially due to weather or permits." The permits portion was a lie, but I wasn't going to throw Sandy under the bus. "I know that doesn't help, but there's nothing I can do. I'm sorry."

She glared at me and then stormed off. Her friend reassured us everything was fine and then followed her. An uncomfortable silence descended on the table.

"Well, that was an awkward way to start the trip," I said, reaching for my cup. "Can someone pass me the wine?"

Everyone broke into laughter and raised their cups in a toast. No one appeared to care about the woman's outburst. If anything, the group seemed closer now. We were halfway through dinner and a second bottle of wine when the two women returned. The angry one stood at the far end of the table and apologized to everyone. She didn't speak to me for the rest of the evening.

Every trip had its difficulties, but angry clients were rare. Even Gregor hadn't seen someone get so upset, let alone within our first hour together. The next three days weren't going to be any easier. Half Dome trips required long days and involved a lot of steep trails. And because Sandy had confused the permits, we needed to take a bus to our trail-head, a bus that ran once a day. If we missed it, the trip was over. So the next morning, once we had woken up and packed our gear and made it to the bus stop, I assumed the worst was behind us.

"Everyone take a few minutes to run to the restroom, please," I shouted to our group. "Let's meet back here in ten minutes." I turned to Gregor. "I'm going to take a leak. I'll be right back."

I dropped my pack and trip paperwork on a nearby step and then went to the bathroom. When I returned, the angry woman was hovering next to my backpack, skimming through the instructions Sandy had given me. She looked at me and then held up the folder and stabbed at the ti-tle page with the same finger from the night before.

"So, I see I've booked the Trainwreck Trip," she said.

Oh, for fuck's sake.

For a moment I considered lying. Then I realized I had nothing to lose and that the best thing to do was to be honest, so I unveiled the en-tire fiasco. I told her about Sandy's mistaken permits and our last-minute plan to use a different trail. I even admitted I'd never seen it before.

"Look," I told her, glancing around at the cliffs and trees. "We're in the most beautiful place in the world, a place very few people ever get to see, and now we get to see a new part of it. I know you're upset we won't be going over Cloud's Rest, but this'll still be an amazing trip. I promise."

The woman didn't say anything. She just sat there watching me with a furrow in her brow as if she were trying to read my mind. Then, after what felt like a minute, she stood and offered me her hand.

"It's not your mistake," she said. "I appreciate you being honest with me. I just hope the rest of the trip goes well."

I didn't have the heart to tell her it was supposed to rain for two days, and that it would probably be too dangerous to hike to the top of Half Dome, not that it would have mattered anyway. Twenty minutes later, before our bus had even left the valley, the rain began. And for the rest of the day, a cold mist fell from the gray clouds that drifted over the pine trees on our way to camp.

It was dusk when we dropped our packs in an ashy clearing near a creek. A fire had burned the area years before and downed trees and blackened manzanita dotted the meadow. It wasn't a particularly pretty place, especially for Yosemite. But that didn't seem to matter to the clients. For them it was special, even with the rain, and that made it special to me.

That evening we all sat around a campfire and ate dinner and talked about what had brought us to Yosemite. Several people said they had never been to California and wanted to learn how to backpack. A few others were Bay Area natives who had never seen the park. One of them, a woman with strawberry blond hair and enormous green eyes, told us she had been born blind and didn't feel safe backpacking alone.

"I had cataract removal surgery when I was three years old," she said. "I used to wear those thick Coke bottle glasses. I wound up getting synthetic lenses when I was nineteen, but I've had a few complications over the years, and I almost lost my sight a few times." She paused and turned to look at the ridgeline near our campsite, with its row of backlit trees standing silhouetted against the moonlight. "It's pretty incredible to finally see this place."

Everyone fell silent. Not an uncomfortable silence, but the silence of people sitting together around a campfire, each of us gazing at the flames or stars. After a moment someone asked, "How did you guys become backpacking guides?" Gregor looked at me. I knew he didn't like talking about himself, so I shared some of my story, mostly about sitting chair in the hospital and the first time I had gone outside, when I stood in the sunlight and listened to the birds and the murmur of cars on the highway. I could have shared some childhood memory about hiking with my dad, but no other experience had ever affected me as deeply as those few minutes on that sidewalk in Texas.

Everyone fell quiet again, but this time the silence seemed awkward. Every cough and whisper sounded louder than before. I was poking at the fire with a stick when the woman with the green eyes spoke to me.

"Thanks for sharing that," she said.

It wasn't the first time I'd told clients about my life. Over the summer, I'd probably shared some part of my story with at least a dozen people. And every time I had, I wondered if I'd done something wrong. Not because they didn't understand, but because they did. Sometimes, usually later and away from people, one of them would walk with me and share a painful memory, and I'd spend the rest of the day feeling like I had reminded them of something they had never wanted to remember. Yet when every trip came to an end, they would embrace me and thank me for being honest. I felt guilty at first. But eventually, after talking to those dozen or so people, I began to feel like sharing my story was part of being a guide.

The following morning we packed our gear and started toward our next campsite, on the shoulder of Half Dome about seven miles away. The first half of the trail wound through a narrow corridor of pine trees before stopping at the top of a ridge that overlooked Little Yosemite Valley. Across the valley, a thousand feet above us, stood the backside of Half Dome. The sky behind it was gray and angry. When the first drops of rain began to fall, I stopped the group and talked to Gregor while everyone took off their packs and put on their rain gear.

"What do you think?" I asked him. "Stop and eat lunch here? Or head down into the valley?"

He looked at the sky. "I'll set up the tarp. Let's eat lunch and wait for a bit. That way if it gets worse, at least they'll be fed."

The rain grew stronger. Everyone dug their lunches out of their packs while Gregor and I strung the tarp between some trees. Then, just as the wind began to pick up, the patter of the rain changed to a soft clicking sound. One of the clients stuck out her hand, and a tiny piece of ice, like rock salt from the sky, bounced off her palm.

"Yay! Hail!" she shouted.

No, no. Not yay. Hail is bad.

A bolt of lightning crackled overhead and struck the top of Half Dome. The thunder was monstrous. For half an hour our group huddled under the tarp, shivering while everyone stared at their soggy lunches, wondering why they had spent hundreds of dollars to eat a cold packet of tuna fish in the rain. It's easy to romanticize backpacking, but the truth is that a good portion of it is no different from life: it's filled with hardship and suffering, until days or weeks or years later when the pain is gone and all that remains are good memories.

The hail slowed and then turned to rain. Gregor stepped out from the shelter and walked toward his pack as if he had forgotten something. He stopped after a few paces and we all turned to watch him. For a moment he just stood there. Then he turned his face to the sky and closed his eyes, his arms outstretched like a shaman communing with a storm.

Gregor was known among the guides as "the guy who loved weather." At one time or another, most of us had seen him jump in a frozen river or run around in the rain. Once, I followed him into a lake, only to turn around when I realized the water was so cold that I could barely breathe. I'd always wondered if he was trying to convince himself of something, that maybe things weren't as bad as they seemed. But that day, as I stood there watching him, instead of thinking of Gregor or the clients, I thought of the hospital and my old roommate Michael.

It was nighttime and the light from the hallway filled our bedroom. Michael was in restraints back then. We had been signing to each other when he stopped and sniffed the air. His eyes grew wide.

"Rain," he signed.

I pointed at my nose and shook my head. Michael gestured to the wall behind him.

"The AC," he whispered.

Every room on the unit had its own window-mounted air conditioner. And while they didn't do much to change the temperature, they did have a vent that opened to the world outside. Michael's bed was nearest the window, and because I was rarely allowed off my chair, I'd forgotten about the vent.

I sat up in bed and glanced at the hallway. The night staff checked our rooms every fifteen minutes, but I couldn't remember the last time I'd seen their shadow pass our door.

"Hurry," Michael whispered.

I jumped out of bed and scurried across the room and hid in the crawl space between his bed and the air conditioner. I hadn't been outside in months. My senses were so hungry that I could smell the wet earth and rain without even opening the vent.

"Open it," Michael whispered.

I searched for the controls and twisted the dial that opened the vent. A cold draft of fresh air blew straight into my face, hard enough that my hair fluttered to the side. I'd forgotten what that felt like. I looked at the hallway one last time before pushing my nose between the slats of the air conditioner and drawing a breath. I must have knelt there for nearly twenty seconds, imagining how it would feel to stand in the courtyard outside our screened window with my face turned to the sky.

The image of Gregor gazing at the heavens reminded me of that night, of the smell of wet grass and leaves and the low growling of thunder in the distance. I had always loved that memory. It felt like such a gift, kneeling there with my nose in an air conditioner, connected to a world that seemed so far away. I don't know how long I stood there watching Gregor. I remember seeing a flicker of lightning and then turning to look at the woman with the green eyes. She smiled.

"What an amazing moment," I said.

The white-haired woman glared at me. The rest of the group just stared at their lunches or Gregor, waiting for the rain to stop. I couldn't help but feel sorry for all of them.

"I know this isn't exactly what you all signed up for," I said, "but there are people who'd do anything to be here right now, but they can't. They're stuck in a hospital or going through chemo or living under a bridge somewhere."

No one said anything. A few people nodded and went back to picking at their lunches. By then the rain had slowed and Gregor returned to the group with a package of Oreos and a stove to make some tea.

"Let's pack up and get going soon," he said. "After a couple of hot drinks and some cookies, we'll all feel better."

The rain continued for the rest of the day. Gregor led the group down a series of switchbacks and into the valley, where we followed the Merced River until we came to the trail that led to our last night's campsite. From the back our group looked like a band of hooded monks walking to a funeral. No one spoke. The only sound was the static of the rain. The storm had passed by the time we got to camp, so Gregor began cooking our dinner while I collected dry bits of tinder from under trees and rocks. Damp wood doesn't burn well, and it produces a lot of smoke, but a fire draws people together, and any good guide knows that the even the most miserable group of folks will throw a party around the tiniest of flames.

An hour later our group sat eating dinner around the campfire. They looked like they had known each other for years, with their jackets and pants and socks draped over logs to dry near the fire. After listening to the rain all day, the world seemed quieter now. The flames popped and crackled while everyone ate in silence.

I'd just started washing our dishes when someone mentioned 9/11. "Today's the tenth anniversary," they said. Everyone fell quiet again. It seemed strange to be in a beautiful place on such a terrible day. A few people shared stories about where they had been when it happened, and eventually someone asked me. I told them about living with Nathan, back when I'd ride my bike to Starbucks and read books and daydream about changing my life.

"I never thought I'd be a guide back then," I said. "And now here I am, doing dishes on the shoulder of Half Dome."

One of the clients, a blond woman whose husband was also on the trip, asked me if I wanted help. I almost said yes. I'd always hated doing dishes. Instead, I sat there with my hands in that pot of soapy water, thinking—for the first time in my life—that I loved serving people.

"No, thanks," I told her. "Tomorrow's my fortieth birthday. I'm just grateful to be here and spend it with all of you."

Everyone made a big deal out of my birthday. It didn't exactly bother me, but my parents had forgotten my birthday so many times that I'd stopped celebrating it. To me it was nothing but a sad reminder of all the years they had never called me, so by the time I'd finished the dishes and the clients had shuffled off to bed, I figured they had forgotten about it too.

The next morning came early. The moon was up when I woke, and the sky was dotted with stars. The only trace of yesterday's rain was the smell of wet earth and wood. I woke the clients while Gregor made a pot of coffee, and after promising everyone a huge breakfast once we returned from the summit, I followed the group as Gregor led the way.

The main trail up Half Dome led to a series of steps chiseled into the granite. The "staircase," as we called it, ascended several hundred feet to a narrow ridgeline at the base of the cables. Often this section of the route was jammed with people waiting to get to the top, but after two days of rain the crowds were gone. Gregor stood at the front of our group, dumb-founded.

"There's no one here," he said. "We're alone."

One of the clients pointed at the dome. "Holy shit. Are we going up those?"

Two cables, placed arm's length apart, climbed the final slope to the summit. Every twenty feet or so, wooden boards were attached to the granite so people could stop and rest. The climb usually took more than an hour because of the crowds. But we were alone that morning, and twenty minutes later we were standing on top, lifting our arms overhead to watch the sun crawl down our fingertips and across the peaks of the high country.

I don't know who began singing first, whether it was Gregor or the woman with the green eyes or one of the other clients, but as I stood there listening to them sing "Happy Birthday," I thought of the first time I met Sandy, when she said that every group of clients would feel like a family. At the time it sounded nice, like something people say only because they want it to be true. But now, on my last trip of the season, I understood. Since the day I'd met Doni and Zach's family, and then Robert and Julie and the kids, it seemed as if fate or the universe had made sure that, in the absence of a birth family, I would always have a chosen family, and that instead of a home or a house, I'd been given the mountains and trees and stars. And now, after becoming a guide in an attempt to leave my past behind, I'd accomplished something far more important. I'd found a purpose. For years I'd hidden from the world. I'd played games and read books instead of giving people another chance. And although I had friends, I didn't trust anyone completely. But when I was guiding, people relied on me. I built their fires and cooked their dinners. I made them hot water bottles in the middle of the night. After months of caring for those people, I realized that nothing mattered more to me than helping them, because once again the universe had given me a family, as long as I had the courage to accept them.

24

A Broken Wind-up Toy

My first season as a guide came to an end with the Trainwreck Trip, and along with it went most everything that brought me happiness. I don't recall much about my last few days in Sonoma or the drive back to Dallas. All I remember are snapshots that seem to symbolize how I felt about leaving California. A cold breakfast buffet in a hotel in Albuquerque. Long stretches of lonely highway. Dust devils drifting across the plains of West Texas. I'm sure I spoke to Dad and Linda before I left, but I have no memory of it. I don't even recall seeing Sandy after the Trainwreck Trip. But I knew I'd see them again. I was a guide now, and soon I would be going back to California and Yosemite. And this time I knew I would stay there forever.

The day after I returned to Texas, I began to pack. Books. DVDs. Tundra's ashes. The one box of Jennifer's belongings I'd kept, filled with a dozen random things including her beer bottle and some postcards she had sent me. Whatever I could replace in California, I gave away. Every item I threw in the trash filled me with joy. I moved in with two friends who lived in a nearby suburb. Two months later I hired a moving company to store all my things until I found a place to live in California. Robert had warned me not to leave Dallas too quickly, to take my time and say goodbye, but now that I had a new life waiting for me, I didn't care. I stripped my existence down to nothing but essentials. I slept on an air mattress and kept my clothing in a suitcase, because in a couple of months I wouldn't live in Texas anymore. I'd finally be free.

It was sometime that November when Robert called me. He told me he'd been in and out of the hospital again, but he was feeling better now. "It's nothing to worry about, Ban," he said. "It's just the same old cellulitis in my legs." He asked about my time in California, and I told him about Yosemite and the clients and the lunch I'd had with my dad when we ordered the same thing.

"I sure bet he's happy to have you back in his life," Robert said.

"I guess. We even talked about the hospital, but he doesn't really like talking about it. He doesn't seem to like talking about anything except his time in the navy."

"I'm sure he still feels guilty about putting you in there," Robert said. "He's not exactly blameless."

I didn't know what to say. After everything Dad and Linda had told me about my mom, I wasn't sure what to believe anymore, and there was no one I could ask to get the truth. And not just about my family but about anything, about the hospital or the doctors or why they had kept me there. I'm sure Robert would have said I never needed to be in the hospital. But without an MRI or an X-ray, like my dad suggested, there didn't seem to be any truth at all.

"I'm moving back to California in a couple of weeks," I said finally.

Robert's voice rose, the way it always did when he was smiling.

"I'm proud of you, son," he told me.

I said, "Thanks," although it was difficult for me to hear the words. I'd never taken compliments well, not after years of feeling like a failure.

"Can I ask you a favor?" Robert said.

"Sure."

"I want you to find a therapist when you settle down out there," he told me, "when you're ready."

He had said the words in a small voice, as if he were asking for forgiveness. The word *therapy* made my stomach turn. I almost started yelling at him.

"Why?" I asked.

"Ban, what you experienced in the hospital was not therapy. That was abuse. Therapy's different. It's a journey. But instead of learning about the mountains, you're learning about yourself. There's a lot of beautiful stuff in there for you to find."

I laughed.

"Will you at least promise to try?" he asked.

No one else could have said those words to me. I trusted Robert and he knew that.

"Yeah, Pop," I said, trying not to sound angry. "I'll go someday. For you. I promise."

I'm not sure why Robert asked me to see a therapist that day. I'd struggled with depression for years and he had never suggested it before. He probably knew I was lonely, and I'm sure he knew that therapy terrified me. But I also knew he was right. The hospital wasn't therapy, and the only way I would ever truly leave the hospital behind me was to give therapy another chance.

The land around Jennifer's grave was not special. Flat and mostly featureless, it contained only a fence, grass, a few trees, and a wide-open sky. I couldn't count how many times I'd been there, through sixteen years of birthdays and anniversaries and sleepless nights. At first it was a terrible place, a land of grief and tears. Slowly, it changed, or I changed, until that grassy meadow became something like a church, a quiet place where her presence could live. Now, after I had built the beginnings of a new life in California, her grave felt like a resting place. Not just for her but also for some part of me that still belonged to her, a part of me I didn't need anymore.

Of course she didn't know that I'd come to say goodbye, or that I was driving to California that morning. But as I knelt in the grass and kissed her gravestone, I pictured her looking up at me, worried, as if she had heard a rumor and now I had to tell her the truth.

"Yeah," I said. "I'm moving. Back to California. But I guess you already know that."

I'd brought a dozen white roses, like I always did, and I fumbled with the cellophane while I wondered what to say. For as long as I could remember, Jennifer's grave had felt like a safe place. Now I felt awkward. I'd never imagined saying goodbye.

"I figured I'd bring these for your birthday, since I'm leaving today," I said. "It's hard to believe you'd be forty next month. I thought I'd bring you roses forever, but it's been so long since you died. I guess I've finally changed."

I was ashamed of admitting that I was different now, that I wanted to live my life without her. I wouldn't have said the words if I'd thought about them first. But as they hung in the air, I realized I *was* different now, that I didn't need to keep holding on to Jennifer anymore.

"You know, as screwed up as we were back then, you're still the best friend I've ever had. I'll always love you. Even after all these years, I still remember a million things about you. The sound of your laugh and the way you'd smile. The way you'd stand on your tiptoes and kiss me. How you used to shave your legs in the pool.

"Maybe that's all heaven is," I said. "When someone only remembers all the good things about you."

I set Jennifer's roses on her gravestone and got to my feet. There were so many things I wanted to say, but I'd said them all before. They didn't need to be said again.

"I'll always love you, Jennifer. I'll miss coming here to see you. Maybe I'll come back someday. Maybe I'll bring my wife and kids, or maybe I'll be a lonely old man. I don't know."

I suppose, on some level, I knew Jennifer wasn't really there, no more than she had been living in the house with me all those years before. Yet whether she was really listening or not didn't matter. All that mattered now was how I felt.

I knelt and kissed her headstone. Then I repeated the last words she had said to me years before.

"Alligator food."

Two days and fourteen hundred miles later, I parked in front of my new apartment in Lafayette, California. I'd only been to the small town once to go on a hike with Sandy, and I'd loved it ever since. It looked like a scene out of a Norman Rockwell painting, with its main street lined with light posts and banners and one small post office. Yosemite was three and a half hours away, and Sandy and Ron lived in the town next door.

Everything seemed fine at first. I got a part-time job at a local REI and sold backpacking gear and taught people about Yosemite. Every week Sandy and Ron would invite me over for dinner and we'd talk about the upcoming guiding season. But eventually the depression I thought I'd left in Dallas found me again, and without a game or a girlfriend or clients to focus on, I felt like a broken wind-up toy, as if something inside me had been twisted too tightly. I began having flashbacks of the hospital, images of the wall in my room and the sound of Sonia shrieking in the distance. Hundreds of memories came flooding back. Sometimes I'd be at the coffee shop or on a date and I'd hear her calling out for help. I felt like I was suffocating. My mind had recorded hundreds of details of the worst moments my life, and now it was replaying them over and over. They weren't like normal memories, little vignettes that I could revisit whenever I wanted. They were entire experiences. The smell of cinnamon disinfectant. The rattling of restraints on Sonia's bed. The way her bloody saliva ran down the walls. Dr. Fisher's stoic expression as she watched the staff roll Sonia into the dayroom like a tranquilized animal. My mind had recorded every detail, and now it was forcing me to relive them whenever it wanted, even when I was standing in line at the grocery store.

After weeks of flashbacks, I found a blog about PTSD and something called "dissociation." Every word seemed to hold some terrible truth about me, about why my memories felt like scenes in a movie. And not just scenes from the hospital but scenes from the rest of my life, like the day

I'd been left at the airport and the morning Jennifer died. Everything I read terrified me. My mind felt defective now, and there didn't seem to be anything I could do to fix it.

Finally, after calling a suicide hotline and hanging up, I called Robert instead.

"Have you tried calling a therapist?" he asked.

I almost lied to him, but I didn't. "No," I said.

"Talk to them over the phone first, Ban. Tell them what happened. If they're a good therapist, they'll understand."

The next day I spent hours searching through dozens of websites and reviews before I called a therapist. She was an older woman with short gray hair and kind brown eyes. I don't know why, but something about her photo made me feel safe, although she was difficult to read over the phone. She didn't sound particularly nice, but she sounded honest. I told her I was interested in seeing a therapist and that I had some concerns. "Why?" she asked. I told her I'd been in a hospital and forced to sit in a chair for hours a day. I told her about Sonia and how she had been tied to her bed for months. I told her I was afraid of being sent to another hospital. She was quiet for a moment.

"You have every reason to be afraid," she said. "It took courage for you to call."

I went to see her later that week. I didn't feel anything akin to therapist first-date fireworks, but I left the room freely and unrestrained and without her threatening to have me signed in to an institution or medicated. Week after week, I'd sit in her office and stare out the window and talk about the hospital. Once, when she began writing in a notepad, I stopped speaking and glanced at her.

"Why did you just look at me?" she asked.

"It scares me when you take notes. I wonder what you're writing, if you think something's wrong with me, like I'm sick. They were always writing in our charts in the hospital."

She set her notepad on the table next to her. "I'll stop. I'm sorry."

I looked away again.

"Would you like to see my notes?" she asked.

"Isn't that unethical or something?"

"They're about you," she said. "There's nothing wrong with you. You're hurt and you came here to talk to me about it."

Something about her kindness made me angry. I didn't want pity, especially from a therapist.

"Why are you so nice to me?" I said. "It didn't take courage for me to call you. I'm not strong. I'm scared, just like I was in the hospital. Back then, all I thought about was me. I was terrified all the time. The whole place became a game to me, even my friends. I just sat there and watched the staff tie them down, over and over."

"Then they would have tied you down, and you knew that," she said. "You knew better. You did the only thing you could. You controlled yourself, even when other people couldn't."

"But I didn't even try to help them," I cried. "I just hid from everything. I thought I'd escaped that place, that I was free. But I'm not. I feel like I'm still there."

Those words haunted me for weeks. Since the day I'd left the hospital, the only thing I'd wanted was to be something other than an ex–psychiatric patient. Now, after years of struggling to build a new life that had nothing to do with that place, here I was, paying a therapist a hundred dollars a week so I could talk about what "therapy" had done to me. I felt humiliated. I imagined what my friends from the hospital would think if they knew I was seeing a therapist. Every Thursday I shuffled out of her office in tears, wondering if I'd made a huge mistake. Half the time I'd sit on the curb behind her building and cry until I was calm enough to walk home.

I don't remember when I first found Sonia, but after joining Facebook and getting friend requests from Nathan and Robert and his partner, Barry, and my friend Jonathan, I realized I might be able to reconnect with my friends from the hospital too. I searched for everyone I could remember from unit C. Many of them had already found one another. Others had died or vanished. But of all those friends, Sonia still haunted me. She looked so different in her pictures on Facebook, outside the walls of the hospital, smiling and free of her restraints.

I must have stared at Sonia's picture for twenty minutes before I wrote her a message. I was still writing an hour later when I deleted it. I wrote another the next day and I deleted that one too. It became part of my routine. Every day I'd walk to the coffee shop and pour my heart out and ask Sonia to forgive me.

"I'm sorry I never helped you," I wrote. "I didn't know what to do. I was so afraid. I didn't want to get put in restraints. But every time I sat there and watched you get rushed, I felt like something inside of me was dying. I'd sit in my room and listen to you fight and scream and I never did anything. I don't know what I could've done to help, but I'm still sorry, Sonia. I'm sorry."

I deleted every message I wrote to her, but I kept writing them anyway. I felt like a coward again. I didn't know what to say to her. Everything I wanted to share sounded so desperate and sad. But instead of finding something else to do, I'd just sit at the coffee shop and open a little door inside me and record everything that came spilling out. Then I'd delete it all and do it again the next day.

I found other friends on Facebook too. Michael lived in Montana, but another friend said he never responded to messages. Sean still lived in Dallas and had a daughter now. The guy who snuck into a girl's bedroom and wound up in restraints had started his own business. When he told me he had dated another girl from the unit years before, I sent her a friend request and she told me never to mention that she'd been in the hospital to anyone.

"I don't want anything to do with that place anymore," she said. "My husband and kids don't even know about it, and I don't want them to ever find out."

By the time guiding season arrived, Robert was sick again. I called to check on him and Barry answered the phone in a whisper and said he was sleeping. "He's getting better though," Barry told me. "Try not to worry." I worried anyway. Barry said he would leave him a message, and when I called again the next day Robert answered on the first ring. I told him I'd found a therapist and he almost dropped the phone.

"I'm so proud of you, son. You have no idea how far you've come," he said. "What's she like?"

"Honest."

Robert chuckled. "Well, that's a first for you, isn't it? An honest therapist."

He groaned as if he were struggling to sit up in bed. He sounded old and tired and something in his voice scared me. I asked how he was feeling and he said, "Fine." I didn't believe him. Robert had told me he was fine more times than I could count, and it usually meant he wasn't fine and didn't want to talk about it.

"Barry and I are taking a road trip soon," he said, changing the subject. "We're driving to Tennessee and Mississippi to go to Natchez Trace. We'll be there around your birthday. I'll have to send you some pictures."

Barry had taken care of Robert for years, and I knew he wouldn't plan a multistate road trip if Robert wasn't doing well. I also knew there was no point in fussing over him, since there was nothing I could do from two thousand miles away.

"Just be careful, okay?" I said.

"Don't worry about me. You've got enough on your plate out there. Speaking of which, what made you find a therapist?"

"I was just lonely. I started dating a lot of people. Then I started having flashbacks."

Robert didn't say anything. He didn't need to. Since the day we'd met, he'd understood me in a way that no one else did. But that day, as I sat there thinking about him lying in bed in Arkansas, all his love and kindness suddenly felt too heavy to bear.

"I know I've told you this a thousand times," I said, my voice trembling. "But there's no way I can ever repay you for everything you've done for me."

"You've already repaid me. You're helping other people now. That's what matters."

I began to cry. I tried to speak, but all that came out was a long stream of gibberish and tears. Maybe it was the weeks of therapy. Or the fact that, for the first time in my life, Robert seemed mortal. But whatever the reason, I was too tired and fragile to be strong anymore, and I lay on the floor next to my sofa and wept.

"Why did I survive?" I cried. "Why didn't Jennifer? Or Kevin? I still hate myself for being alive when they're dead."

"You can't blame yourself for surviving. There are so many things that make up who we are. Our nature, our families, our friends and experiences. Even simple luck. And in all those things, you wound up with something very rare, and now you're sharing it with others. Who knows how many lives you'll change someday?"

I sat up and leaned against the sofa and wiped my eyes.

"Thanks, Pop," I said. "I love you."

"I know you do, Ban. I love you too. I'll give you a call once we're home from our trip, okay? Try not to worry."

I told him I wouldn't worry even though I would. Then he hung up.

25

He Loved You

Throughout most of my life, depression had driven me inward, away from people and the world outside. Now it drove me toward them. Halfway through backpacking season, I was working six days a week, either guiding for Sandy or helping customers at REI. My one free day was dedicated to therapy and laundry and organizing my backpacking gear. My only time alone was at night. And when I wasn't guiding, I spent my evenings looking through all the photographs I'd taken throughout the summer.

I don't recall being unhappy back then, at least not when I was working. Even in retrospect, I remember those times fondly. I liked who I'd become. Therapy wasn't miserable anymore and my flashbacks were mostly gone. And I still loved being a guide. Every week I met new people, and I made a difference in their lives, just like Robert had hoped.

But soon September arrived and with it came our last trip of the season. REI had asked Sandy to create a new trip for people who were interested in a more glamorous camping experience, or what came to be known as "glamping." Sandy thought it was the stupidest thing she had ever heard of.

"But if I don't do it," she said, "REI will find another contractor who will."

Days later Sandy unveiled the "Lodge Trip," a weeklong series of day hikes based out of Yosemite Valley. Everything was provided. Hotel rooms in Yosemite Lodge, meals, snacks, even a chartered bus. All the clients had to bring was clothing. We'd even meet them at the airport and take the bus to the valley. From the day she conceived it, the Lodge Trip represented everything Sandy hated about Yosemite. We wouldn't be backpackers. We'd be tourists, no different from the millions of other people who came to the park every year.

For six days Sandy and I met the clients outside their rooms at the lodge. Then we'd eat breakfast in the cafeteria and guide the group on a day hike around the valley. Until that week, Yosemite had been something like a church to us, with its stone walls and ceiling made of stars and sky. Now it felt empty. I lost count of how many times Sandy pulled me aside and pointed at the peaks in the distance. "We belong out there," she'd say. "Not here with all the tourists." We hadn't made it halfway through the week when Sandy said she'd never run the trip again.

"Let REI find someone else who wants to do their fucking glamping trips," she told me. "I can't do another one. I'm a backpacker, not some diva who needs a shower every night."

The last full day of the Lodge Trip fell on a Saturday, three days after my birthday. And because cell phone coverage was poor in the valley, the birthday texts and voicemails trickled in for days. I didn't usually pay much attention to my phone when I was guiding. But when I never heard from Robert, I began to worry.

Sandy and I cooked breakfast for the clients that morning at a row of picnic tables near the lodge. After cleaning up and hauling all the gear back to her room, we guided our group to the top of Yosemite Falls, following a seven-mile-long trail that rose 2,700 feet from the valley floor. I checked my phone every time the clients stopped for water or pictures. We were at the top of the falls and halfway through lunch when my phone finally buzzed. Barry had called me twice. He didn't leave a message.

A wave of nausea rose in my throat. Sandy walked over and put her hand on my shoulder.

"Everything okay?" she asked.

"I guess. I don't know. Barry called me a little while ago."

Sandy knew Robert had been sick. "Do you need to call him back?"

"No, it's okay," I lied. "They're taking a road trip in a couple of days. They probably just called to wish me a happy birthday."

We both knew Barry hadn't called to wish me a happy birthday, but I didn't know what else to say. I was afraid something had happened, but admitting it would have made it impossible to bear. So instead I wandered behind the group for the rest of the day, holding that fear inside me like a moth in a jar.

It was midafternoon when we parted ways with the clients outside the lodge. Sandy followed me to my room and I sat on the foot of my bed and stared at my phone.

"I can leave if you want," she said.

I shook my head and she sat next to me while I dialed Barry's number. I could hear my heart beating in my ears. He answered a moment later. He had been crying.

"Hi, Barry."

"Hello," he said.

"I saw that you called. We were out with the clients. I'm sorry."

"That's okay." He was quiet for a long time. "Robert died this morning."

I almost said, "I know." Sandy put her arm around me. I felt like I was outside my body, watching over her shoulder.

"He saved my life," I said.

"He loved you, Banning."

I began to cry. My tears felt small and feeble, tiny in comparison with the monstrous grief trying to claw its way out of me. I tried to cry harder, but it only made me stop.

"I know he loved me," I said. "I loved him too. I wouldn't be here without him."

Barry was quiet again. "I'll call you soon, once we have a date for the funeral."

"I love you," I said.

"I love you too, Banning."

I hung up and set the phone beside me. Sandy leaned over and gave me a hug. I felt her arms around me, so different from Robert's. It reminded me of the day he'd found me standing in my old room in the hospital years before, when he performed his exorcism, holding me in an awkward bear hug with his salt-and-pepper hair in my face.

Sandy gave me a final squeeze. I stood and walked to the window and looked outside, at the cliffs and spires that lined the valley. I kept trying to cry but nothing came out, so I leaned my forehead against the window and imagined Robert standing next to me, telling me everything would be okay like he had so many times before.

———

The rest of the Lodge Trip passed in a blur. I remember drinking three glasses of bourbon at the bar that night and then saying goodbye to the clients at the airport the next afternoon. Sandy drove us home while I stared out the window. I don't recall saying anything to her. I don't even remember driving home from her house. I only remember dropping my pack on the floor of my tiny apartment and then showering in the dark, still too shocked to cry more than a few small tears.

I didn't attend Robert's funeral. Flights were expensive and I couldn't afford to take time off from work, or at least that's what I told my therapist. After Robert's death, I spent most of our sessions telling her stories about him, about the lawsuit and the years afterward when the doctors sued us. Soon she began asking how I felt, and I'd say something like "I'm sad" or "I miss him." Then she'd arch an eyebrow and sit back in her chair and look at me. I didn't know how to answer her. I'd known Robert for twenty years. He had saved my life. How could I explain that in a bunch of forty-five-minute sessions?

"You know, he's the one who asked me to find a therapist," I told her. "He made me promise."

"Why did he ask you to find a therapist?" she said.

"He said what I'd experienced in the hospital wasn't therapy. It was abuse. He said therapy was an adventure, like wandering through the mountains." I laughed. "I don't even know why I come here sometimes. All I do is cry. It's almost like he knew he was going to die and that I'd need someone else to talk to. And now, after months of my talking about the hospital and Jennifer, now he's dead."

I don't know why saying those words suddenly made Robert's death seem more real. But the moment they left my mouth, something gave way and all the tears I'd been holding inside me finally came pouring out. My therapist sat quietly with her hands in her lap, watching me while I wept. I felt like a child. She handed me a box of tissue and I set it next to me and turned and looked out the window.

"I don't know what I'm supposed to do now," I cried. "I wouldn't even be here if it weren't for him. I would have killed myself years ago. And now he's gone."

My therapist leaned forward, as if to emphasize her words. "Robert may have helped you, but you did the work."

"I told you before," I said, raising my voice. "It wasn't courage or strength that saved me. It was fear. I didn't survive the fucking hospital or Jennifer's death because I'm strong. I survived because I was too afraid to kill myself."

"A lot of survivors feel that way."

"God, I hate that fucking word. I'm not a survivor. I was just scared. I'm still scared."

"You survived the hospital and Jennifer's death because you worked your ass off," she said. "And now you're here in my office, working your ass off again. You might have been scared, but no one forced you to come see me. You called because you're strong enough to ask for help."

I wanted to scream at her. I refused to accept that I was stronger than some of my friends who had been in the hospital, especially Jennifer and Kevin.

"So what am I supposed to do now?" I said. "Robert's dead. I can't repay him for everything he did for me."

"Can't you, though? What do you think he'd want you to do?"

I sank into the sofa and dug my palms into my eyes. "He'd want me to keep guiding, I guess. He'd want me to keep helping people."

With guiding season over, I began working nearly forty hours a week at REI. Everyone at the store knew me as "the backpacking guide" or "the guy who worked in Yosemite." To them, I was just a tall, skinny guy who knew a lot about sleeping bags and how to shit in the woods. What my coworkers didn't know was that being a guide was the only thing that really mattered to me, especially now that Robert had died.

It was Halloween when I walked into work dressed as the main character from *Archer,* complete with a pair of aviator sunglasses and a bushy seventies mustache. I had always loved Halloween. It wasn't a family holiday. There were no gift exchanges or sit-down meals, only kids and candy and people dressed in costumes. Everyone at work was in a good mood that day. Even the break room seemed happy, its walls decorated with smiling skeletons and jack-o'-lanterns.

I was halfway through my shift when my phone rang. We weren't allowed to call or text anyone unless we were on a break, but it was a slow night, so I stepped behind a backpack display and checked my phone. Sandy had called. She and Ron probably wanted to see if I could join them for dinner. Since the day Robert died, they had gone out of their way to spend time with me.

Half an hour later I clocked out for lunch and stepped into the break room to call Sandy. She answered on the first ring. She didn't say anything. For a moment I thought she was crying.

"I'm so sorry," she said.

My heart began to race. "Sorry for what? What's wrong? What happened?"

She fell quiet again. "I lost the contract. They found someone else to run our trips."

The break room seemed to turn sideways. I leaned against the wall next to the sink and then sat down. My body felt too heavy to move.

"I don't understand," I said. "What do you mean?"

"I'm so sorry, Banning. You moved out here to guide for me and now it's all over. They fired me."

Sandy hung up in tears. I wandered out of the break room and finished my shift in a daze. That evening I drove home and spoke to Robert as if he were sitting in the passenger seat. I imagined him smoking his pipe and listening to me while I leaned on the steering wheel and stared at the highway.

"No one will ever hire me as a guide again, Pop," I said to him. "Most guides have years of experience. Sandy only hired me because she's nice."

I'd thought I would work for Sandy for the rest of my life. I'd given away or sold most of what I owned so I could move back to California and live near her and Ron and Yosemite. Now, eight months later, Robert was dead and Sandy had lost her contract. I suppose somewhere in the back of my mind I knew I'd been through worse, but something about losing guiding seemed unfathomable. I'd finally found the one thing I wanted to do with my life. And now, after everything I'd overcome, it had been taken away from me.

Sandy called me the next morning. She blamed herself for everything. I wanted to be angry at her, but she had given me two of the most incredible years of my life. How could I not be grateful for that? Sure, maybe she could have been more cooperative about the Lodge Trip, but then she would have been someone else, someone with different priorities who never would have hired me in the first place.

My first instinct was to move back to Dallas. God knows why. It was the last place I wanted to live, but now California only reminded me of guiding and Yosemite. Every time someone at work asked me about the park, I wanted to crawl into a hole and die. I felt like a failure. When I began having anxiety attacks at work, I asked my manager if I could take a few days off. The next afternoon I reached out to my old friend Jonathan. We hadn't spoken much since I'd moved to California, and his voice reminded me of the day we'd met in the parking lot near my old house, when he stayed with me and Nathan and told us stories about living in his van. I had barely managed to tell him about Sandy and the contract when he interrupted me.

"Dude, don't fucking tell me you're thinking about moving back to Texas."

"But why would I stay here?" I said. "I came out here to be a guide."

"Then find another way to do it, man. You've been through worse. You can't give up now."

I wasn't sure if I'd ever be a guide again, but I knew he was right. If I could survive the hospital and Jennifer's death and still build a new life, then I was strong enough to build another one.

That winter Sandy disbanded her guiding company. She burned all the paperwork and then drove to Yosemite and buried the ashes in the woods. Every time I went to see her, she looked like she hadn't slept in weeks. The few times we went for a walk, she hardly spoke. She would just lumber along next to me and stare at the ground, her head bent forward like a wounded animal's.

I stayed in Lafayette, probably because waiting for things to get better had always worked for me in the past. Besides, I didn't hate therapy anymore. I knew it was helping me. I had friends at work too. I even called my dad sometimes. How would Robert feel if I ruined all those things now? Maybe living my life was all he wanted for me anyway. Maybe I didn't need to help other people to pay him back.

A year after Sandy lost the contract, my manager at REI called me into his office. I'd worked at the store for nearly two years and now most people knew me as "the guy who used to work in Yosemite." I didn't dislike the title. I wore it as a sort of badge of honor. I still backpacked there. And although I wasn't a guide anymore, it still felt like my home.

"What do you know about REI Outdoor School?" my manager asked me.

I told him I knew the name and that I'd heard it was a small group of employees who taught outdoor skills like navigation and mountain biking.

"Well, they're expanding their program," he said, "and they're looking for a backpacking instructor."

I must have sat there for five seconds, staring at him with my mouth half open.

"In Yosemite?" I asked.

He hooked his thumb at the wall. "In Point Reyes, I think, out on the coast."

I applied for the job the next day. Two weeks later they asked me to come in for an interview, so I pulled on a pair of jeans and a T-shirt and drove to the REI in Berkeley. Every employee knew that anyone who dressed up for an interview never got hired. We weren't corporate robots in suits and ties. We thrived outdoors. We had dirty fingernails and spent our paychecks on sleeping bags and climbing gear. I strolled into the store and went upstairs and walked into a tiny room filled with racks of clothing. The regional manager for Outdoor School grinned at me and stood up from behind a table and shook my hand. We chatted for a few minutes before he began asking me questions about backpacking and navigation.

"Can you teach me to use a map and a compass?" he asked.

"You don't know how?"

He chuckled. "No, I know how, but I want you to teach me anyway." He set a map on the table and unfolded it and then handed me a compass.

I spent twenty minutes walking him through topographic maps and contour lines and declination. I was in the middle of a sentence when he pushed the map to the side and looked at me for a few seconds.

"Why do you want to help people get outside?" he asked.

I watched him for a moment. I'd only known him for a few minutes, but something about the way he sat there looking at me with a smile on his face told me that he wanted a real answer, not a safe one.

"I wasn't allowed to go outside for a while when I was teenager," I said, looking away. "I had to sit in a chair and face a wall for a long time. But when I started guiding in Yosemite, I realized the only thing that makes me happier than being outside is helping other people get outside."

He didn't respond. He just sat there, smiling, his eyes seeming to wander through some old memory, as if he were trying to imagine what the outdoors meant to me. After a while he stood and shook my hand, and we chatted for a moment before he walked me to the door.

"Thanks again for coming out today," he said. "You'll hear back from us in a few weeks."

He called me a week later. I thought he was going to ask for a second interview, but he didn't. I already had the job.

26

It Wasn't Your Fault

oint Reyes National Seashore is nothing like Yosemite. It's a lush green peninsula covered in fir trees and lined with beaches. There are no open fields of granite or jagged peaks. Instead there's mist and fog and trees cloaked in moss, like a haunted forest in a storybook. At night, the only sign of the beach is the distant murmur of the waves.

It was just after sunrise when I pulled into a grassy parking lot a few miles away from the beach. I'd worked for Outdoor School for a year and a half, and I'd settled into my life in Lafayette. I still saw my therapist once a week. And after wandering through a series of chaotic relationships, I had begun dating a woman who worked at REI and we'd eventually moved in together. For the first time in my life, I wasn't only happy; I was content. By then I'd run dozens of backpacking trips in Point Reyes. I wasn't a guide anymore. I didn't patch blisters in the rain or make margaritas using snow. I was an instructor now. I taught people how to do those things. I didn't do it for them.

REI provided me with a van and all the gear I'd need to teach the classes. And because most people worked five days a week, our hike followed a short trail to a nearby campsite where we spent just one night. It was an entirely different experience from guiding. There was so much to teach that I often spoke the entire time, even while we were hiking to camp. When we said our goodbyes thirty hours later, I was usually hoarse and exhausted and still three hours away from home.

Before meeting the students, all I knew about them were their names and ages and why they had decided to take the class. It was one of the questions they had been asked when they registered online. Some people said they had never slept in a sleeping bag. Others hadn't backpacked in twenty years. But one common answer always resonated with me: "I want to backpack, but I'm afraid. I don't know what to do." I understood those people. Years before I pulled into that grassy parking lot, I'd written to Sandy and said the same thing.

I was still unloading the van when the students began to arrive. It was the same routine every week. The introverts would park at the far end of the lot and then stare at their phones or dashboards and wonder what they had gotten themselves into. The extroverts would grin at me before they even opened their doors. Then they would hop out of their cars and shake my hand and start asking questions. It never got old.

The first person to arrive that morning parked at the far end of the lot. He must have sat in his car for five minutes before he finally got out. He looked to be about my age. And like me, he was tall and thin, and he walked slowly, watching the ground in front of him as if his mind were somewhere else.

"I'm guessing you're our instructor for the weekend?" he said, shaking my hand.

"Yeah, that's me. My name's Banning. It's nice to meet you."

"Likewise. I'm Ethan." He turned to look at the road as another student arrived. "Hey, my son's driving from downtown. This is kind of a father-son trip for us, but he's running a little late. Is that gonna be a problem?"

A father-son trip, I thought. I couldn't help but like him.

"Don't worry," I said. "I'll get him caught up once he gets here. We'll probably start in about twenty minutes, but we'll be here in the parking lot for at least an hour or two."

Ethan's son arrived a few minutes late. By the time he had gathered his gear and joined us, we were standing in a circle near the van. I always taught the class alone. And after years of guiding for Sandy and teaching for REI, I'd introduced myself to so many people that it felt like a script now.

"Good morning, everyone," I said. "My name's Banning Lyon and I'll be your instructor for the weekend. Before we get started, I'd like to have you all introduce yourselves and share a little about why you're here today, especially since we're going to be stuck together for"—I glanced at my watch—"about thirty hours or so."

Everyone laughed. It was the same awkward laughter I'd heard since my first trip in Yosemite with Sandy four years before. I knew most people were reluctant to spend a night in the woods with strangers. I also knew our first few minutes together were the most important, so I always introduced myself first.

"I've been an instructor for REI for a year and a half now," I said. "Before that, I was a backpacking guide in Yosemite National Park. But about fifteen years ago, I'd never even been there. I lived in Texas. I was a computer gaming addict and a recluse. I hadn't backpacked since I was about ten years old, so don't think I'm special because I'm standing up here teaching. A few years ago, it was my dream to take a class like this."

There was silence. No one said a word. A few people looked at each other and began to laugh. Then Ethan raised his hand.

"What part of Texas?" he asked.

"Dallas. Fort Worth. Austin. I moved around a lot."

"I used to live in Fort Worth too, when I was younger," he said, looking at his son.

I didn't think much of it at the time. After all, it wasn't that rare to meet someone who had lived in Texas. Ten minutes later, once everyone had finished their introductions, I'd forgotten Ethan even mentioned it.

"One of the first things I learned as a guide," I said, "is that I don't actually teach backpacking. All of you already know how to walk around with something heavy on your back. I don't have to teach you how to do that. But it requires a lot of gear, and it's pretty expensive. So why would anyone *want* to do it?"

Silence again. A few people shrugged. Finally someone said, "To go somewhere you can't go in a car?"

"Exactly. And backpacking's not easy. It's really miserable sometimes, actually. I still have days where I wish I could just go home and have a hot shower instead of walking around with a bunch of crap on my back. But then I get to camp and I sit down with my friends and eat some dinner, and I stare at the mountains and think, *Okay, I'm kind of a badass.*"

Everyone laughed again. Everyone always did. Every time.

"All right," I said, pointing at the gear I had piled next to the van. "Let's learn what all this stuff does. Then we'll figure out what we need, what we don't need, and how to pack it. Then we'll hike to camp and have dinner and talk about stoves and water filters and how to take a dump in the woods."

By noon we had packed our things and started for our campsite. Everyone was quiet at first. They didn't know each other yet, and unlike clients on a four-day guided trip, they wouldn't have many opportunities. It wasn't until we stopped to rest at the top of a bluff that everyone began to relax and talk to one another. When someone asked me how I had gone from being a recluse to being a backpacking instructor, all I said was "It's a pretty long story." I didn't mind talking about my past anymore, but I still had a lot to teach before dinner, so I put the story off for later.

The sun was low when we dropped our packs at camp, in the middle of a clearing overlooking the ocean. After organizing all the gear we had carried from the parking lot, I prepped the stoves and fetched some water before helping everyone assemble their tents. No fires were allowed at the campsite. Instead, two picnic tables served as the kitchen, along with a large metal box that prevented animals from getting into our food. It wasn't the most beautiful campsite. But between the moonlight and the fog and the sound of the surf, to the students it must have seemed like paradise.

That evening we sat at the picnic tables and cooked dinner. I was tired of talking, so I sat at the far end of one of the benches and ate quietly while everyone chatted about their jobs and families. It was still overwhelming for me, listening to four or five conversations at once. But after years of practice I'd learned to tune it out most of the time.

"So how'd you go from being a recluse to a backpacker?" someone asked.

I laughed. I always laughed when people asked about my life. They had no idea what I was about to tell them. I felt like someone hiding inside a birthday cake at a party, waiting to jump out and surprise everyone.

"It's a long story," I said again.

Another voice chimed in. "It's not like we're going anywhere."

"It's pretty intense," I added.

"We're adults," someone else said. "I think we can take it."

Over the next half an hour, I told them everything, from my parents' divorce to the hospital to the lawsuit and Robert's death. When I finished, no one spoke. The only sound was the distant rhythm of the surf. I remember turning to look at the ocean and imagining I was still in the hospital, rocking my chair and gazing out the window.

"Sometimes I forget how lucky I am to come out here and do stuff like this," I said. "Sometimes I take it for granted. Then something happens and I remember it all again. There are people out there, right now, who would do anything to be here." I turned back to look at the group. "There's going to come a day when you swear you'll never go backpacking again. You'll be stuck in the rain or a cloud of mosquitoes and you'll wonder why you ever took this class. But if there's anything I want you to remember from this weekend, it's this: our worst day outdoors is way better than our best day without freedom."

Everyone remained quiet. The surf whispered in the distance. One of the students had their headlamp on, and they turned it off and looked at the sky. Then someone spoke from the darkness. It was Ethan.

"You said the hospital was in Dallas," he said.

I nodded.

"What part?"

"Farmers Branch, right next to 635," I said. "It was a big brick building, but it's gone now."

For a moment I wondered if he had ever driven past it. Then he furrowed his brow as if he had never heard of the place. Someone thanked me for sharing my story. Everyone else nodded in agreement. Ethan stood and shook my hand. "Yeah, thanks for sharing that," he said. Soon the group scattered into a dozen shadowy figures, all of them crawling into their tents and zipping up their sleeping bags before drifting off to sleep.

We woke the next morning and made breakfast. I spent an hour teaching everyone how to use a map and compass while we drank our coffee and warmed ourselves in the sunlight. After disassembling our tents and packing our gear, we made our way back to the parking lot on the same trail we had taken the day before. I hiked at the back of the group, listening to people complain about having to go home. It happened every weekend. By the time we reached the cars, everyone wanted to turn around and spend another week in the woods.

We set our packs near the van and I gathered everyone in a circle. It was a tradition I had learned from Sandy, to always thank everyone for sharing their time with me, and for having the courage to spend the weekend with a bunch of strangers. One of the students ran over and gave me a hug. "Thanks again for sharing your story," she said. I lived for those moments. They always left me feeling like my life had finally amounted to something. Soon we all said our goodbyes and promised to keep in touch. Then, once everyone had returned to their cars, I sat in the passenger seat of the van and wrote a summary of the trip for my supervisor.

I had just finished my paperwork when I noticed Ethan standing next to his car. His son had left and he was staring at the grass. I was about to ask him if he needed help when he began walking toward me.

"I was just wondering if you lost something," I said. "Everything okay?"

He stopped a couple of feet away from me. "You said that hospital was in Dallas."

"Yeah, right next to the highway."

"Did they have one in Fort Worth too?" he asked.

I paused. "Yeah, I think so."

"What was it called?"

"Arborfield," I said. "I had a friend who went there."

I thought Ethan was going to pass out. He took an uneasy step forward and then leaned against the side of the van. Then he closed his eyes.

"I was fourteen when they put me in restraints," he said.

The next few moments were blurry. I propped myself against the door of the van and Ethan took a step backward and watched me, waiting for me to do something, to fix what I had done. But there was nothing I could do. He had come here to spend a weekend with his son, only to have me tear open a wound he had probably spent years trying to heal. I felt like I'd ruined his life.

"I've never told anyone," he said, his eyes filling with tears. "But when I heard your story last night, I couldn't sleep, so I told my son." He covered his face with his hands. "I thought that place was behind me. I thought it was all over."

It had been nearly thirty years since the day I left the hospital, when I stood outside the doors of the unit and looked through the windows at my friends still locked inside. Since that day, I had lived a dozen lifetimes. I had survived two lawsuits. I had fallen in love with Jennifer and spent countless nights praying at her altar, a dusty bathroom countertop covered with her clothing and candles. I had lost one father and found another, only to watch him slowly disintegrate after giving his life to save me and a handful of kids who had been locked in the hospital. But Ethan had never experienced any of those things. He had never been a part of our lawsuit. He had never walked through the empty units and stared at the faded outlines of his past. Instead, Ethan had spent decades suffering in silence, struggling to understand the same disaster that Robert had committed his life to helping me overcome.

Six years had passed since Robert died, when I walked to the window of my room in Yosemite Lodge and imagined him telling me that everything would be okay. I held on to those words for months, repeating them over and over until the sound of his voice became as familiar as my own. But now, as I stood in that grassy parking lot and watched Ethan cry into his empty hands, I heard more than Robert's voice. I felt him standing near me again, reminding me of something he had told me so many times before.

"You didn't deserve what happened to you, Ethan," I said. "It wasn't your fault."

Epilogue

Shortly after I finished writing the first draft of this story, my dad was diagnosed with cancer. By then we had built the foundation of a stable relationship. We spoke several times a year. We called each other on our birthdays. Sometimes I drove to Sonoma and spent time with him and Linda. But despite everything we had built, or maybe because of it, I was too afraid to ask him to read my story. I didn't want to ruin our relationship.

One afternoon, when I mentioned it to my therapist, she said, "Isn't that the point of having a relationship? To do something meaningful?" I spent the next few months trying to summon the courage to share my story with my dad. I'd never told him about Robert and Julie and the adoption. He hardly knew anything about Jennifer. He didn't know my mom had hit me and abandoned me. I had no idea how he would react. So after convincing myself to give him a copy, I was shocked when he called me two days later and said he had already finished reading it.

"What did you think?" I asked, my heart crawling up my throat.

He was quiet for a moment. After what felt like a minute, he said, "I'm really grateful you had Robert. I'm glad he loved you so much. I'm sorry he's gone now."

I broke down in tears. Those words were the greatest gift my dad could have given me. His acknowledgment of what Robert meant to me was better than an apology, because he was grateful to Robert even when it meant recognizing his own failure.

My dad died recently, and I often reflect on what my life would have been like if I had never moved back to California to become a guide and rebuild a relationship with him. I never would have walked into REI and met the beautiful woman who would become my wife. I never would have asked her to join me and Sandy and a group of our friends on a backpacking trip into the eastern Sierra, and I never would have hidden her engagement ring in a pair of my socks and proposed to her on the shore of a moonlit lake at twelve thousand feet, surrounded by our friends. We never would have laughed and cried through countless sleepless nights after our daughter was born. We never would have taken her to Yosemite. I never would have become a backpacking guide. And I never would have met Ethan.

Throughout my twelve years as a guide, dozens of clients have asked me, "Would you change anything about your life?" Of course there are things I would change. I would save Jennifer and Kevin and Robert. I would speak up for Sonia and my other friends who were restrained and mistreated. I wouldn't have waited to reach out to my dad. The list is endless. But to change any of those events would have prevented today from happening, and today is a very different place than I ever could have imagined. I'm fifty-one now. I'm a husband. I change diapers and laugh with my wife over videos of our daughter talking to her stuffed animals. I've even stayed in touch with Ethan, and we've exchanged emails and he's thanked me for helping him. I wouldn't trade today for a different past.

I didn't always care about my future, though. For years I lived my life facing backward, searching through the wreckage to try to understand what happened to me, until I'd grown so attached to my memories that I couldn't tolerate living in the present. The past was predictable and familiar. It contained Jennifer and Robert and my unbroken family. It was a snow globe that never dimmed or changed, filled with all the things I had ever loved. Of course, it contained pain as well. But after years of reliving my past, the idea of living without pain terrified me. Who would I be without it?

It wasn't until I moved back to California and became a guide that I began living in the present. My therapist often reminds me that my past will always be there, that I can go and find my snow globe and revisit Jennifer and Robert whenever I miss them. But rebuilding my life has been a slow and messy process. I can't say that I love therapy, but it's enabled me to see a future filled with things that I had thought were impossible. I've rebuilt a relationship with my sister Adrienne. I've reunited with my adopted mom, Julie, and my brothers David and Paul. I still talk to my mom, and she still tells me stories about how wonderful I was when I was a child. And Linda and Emily are still a part of my life.

But scattered among everything I've accomplished are fears that I'm still struggling to understand. Since the day my parents left me at the airport, I've been terrified of being abandoned. The rest of my life only reinforced that fear. Everything from my mom's abuse and neglect to Jennifer's death supported my belief that I would always be alone. So I hid from everyone. Not just in a house but inside myself. I withdrew and dissociated, returning to the quiet place inside me that I'd found so many years ago. It's taken years of therapy and building relationships for me to understand that my old reality is not my new one. And while my goal is to live in the present, it's still difficult for me not to live in the past.

There is no finish line for healing. Therapy, like happiness, is a process, not a fixed point in time. I have good days and bad days. I still struggle. But I look forward now, not backward. And with each passing day, I make myself a better person.

Does that mean I'm grateful for all the things that have made my life possible? No. I'm not. I'm not grateful that Jennifer is dead, or that Sonia spent months of her life strapped to a bed. I'm not grateful for what my parents and the hospital did to me, even though it's given me a deeper appreciation for my life. But I am profoundly grateful for the people who have loved and supported me. Yes, I've worked hard. And yes, I'm still learning to give myself credit for some of the things that I've accomplished. But I am also the product of the kindness of others. And the idea that I, or anyone, can survive trauma and abuse through hard work alone is naive. I needed support. I will always need support. No amount of hard work can replace the love and compassion I've received from others, or the endless beauty of the home that I've found outdoors.

AUTHOR'S NOTE

This story is not intended to discredit or demonize therapy, nor is it anything other than a reflection of my life and experiences. It's my hope that readers walk away from these pages with more compassion for themselves and others, and a deeper understanding of what it's like to survive trauma and abuse. I also hope this story inspires people to spend more time outside, and to discover places that feel important to them. There are countless parks, from local to national, that are waiting to be explored. And like people, they all need support. Yosemite is only one of them.

Acknowledgments

It's impossible to properly express my profound gratitude to the people who supported me in writing this book. Without the encouragement of those mentioned here, and many not mentioned, I never would have completed this story.

Thank you first to my incredible wife, Regina. She was the first person to read my manuscript, over hundreds of mornings of editing my work before going to work for the day. During the six years it took me to write my memoir, throughout countless days of fear and doubt, she believed in me when I didn't have the strength to believe in myself. These words would not exist without her love and compassion. Thank you, Regina.

Jonathan Eig encouraged me to write this story. Without his frequent help and guidance, I never would have found a home for my manuscript. His firm belief that I would eventually succeed gave me the courage to continue forward, even in the face of the inevitable rejections that are part of finding both an agent and a publisher.

ACKNOWLEDGMENTS

My deepest gratitude to my brilliant agent, Meg Thompson, for her passion and wisdom. Since our first meeting online, she has always been there for me, willing to share an expert eye or words of encouragement. Her unwavering kindness and commitment to me and my story have changed the course of my life. I will be forever grateful for the day we first spoke. Thank you for believing in me, Meg.

I would also like to thank Maisa Nammari for digging my manuscript out of Meg's slush pile. Thank you, Maisa!

To my editors, Matt Klise, Meg Leder, and Isabelle Alexander, I owe my heartfelt thanks. Each of you treated me and the people and events in this story with an immense amount of compassion and respect. It was a joy and privilege to work with each of you. Thank you.

I'm also deeply grateful to Maria Shriver for believing in the value of my story. Without her support and unwavering belief in the power of hope and compassion, this book never would have been made.

To Matt Roeser and Jason Ramirez, thank you for creating the incredible cover that embraces these pages. I couldn't have wished for a more beautiful image.

Thank you also to Linda Friedner, Randee Marullo, Tricia Conley, Shelby Meizlik, Mary Stone, and the rest of my team at Penguin Random House.

For their expert knowledge, I would like to thank Clive Matson and his workshop, and Toni Mudgett for her valuable feedback. For their kindness and support, my deepest thanks go out to Ma and Pa McCoy, Nathan McCoy, Chad Cline and Leslie Patrick, Diana and Sprudel, Dr. Ann Steiner, Susan Shapiro, Allison Klein, Jane Durkin, Karen and Rick Najarian, Mike and Becky Duret, Bob and Karen Turner, Gary and

ACKNOWLEDGMENTS

Mariya Croshal, Jonathan Christopher Roberts, and Max Buschini and Kiley Fillinger.

Last, my eternal gratitude to my dearest friends from the hospital who suffered through multiple readings of this story to help me verify some of the events. I will love you all forever.

An incredible memoir about one man's journey to heal from trauma through chosen family, friendship, and nature

AN OPEN FIELD PUBLICATION FROM MARIA SHRIVER

Banning Lyon was an average fifteen-year-old living in Dallas, Texas. He enjoyed skateboarding, listening to punk rock, and even had a part-time job. But in January 1987 his life quickly changed when a school guidance counselor falsely believed he was suicidal after he gave away his skateboard. Days later he was admitted into a psychiatric hospital, and what he was told would be a two-week stay turned into 353 days that would change his life forever.

Banning takes readers through his fraught relationship with his family, the mistreatment he suffered at the hospital, the lawsuit against the owners of the facility, and his desire to make sense of what happened to him. We witness Banning navigate the difficult landscape of trauma and his daily battle to live a normal life. After years of highs and lows that include being adopted by his lawyer and mentor, falling in love and then grieving the death of his fiancée, and being sued by the same doctors who mistreated him, Banning decides to take control of his life and finds hope in the backcountry of Yosemite National Park, where he discovers new purpose in being a backpacking guide. Through friendship, nature, and eventually giving therapy another chance, Banning summons the courage to keep moving forward.

The Chair and the Valley is a raw, gut-wrenching, and amazing story about healing from trauma and starting over. It is a testament to the importance of chosen family, the restorative power of nature, and the strength it takes to build a new life in the face of fear and doubt.

Banning Lyon is a backpacking guide, an instructor, and a public speaker. He currently lives in Martinez, California, with his wife and daughter.

Print and online reviews and features • TV, radio, and podcast interviews • Buzz-building social media campaign • VIP and influencer outreach and activations • Consumer giveaways • banninglyon.com, BanningWrites

For publicity information, please contact Shelby Meizlik at (212) 366-2754 or at smeizlik@penguinrandomhouse.com.

On sale June 4, 2024

The Chair and the Valley is coming in hardcover from The Open Field/Penguin Life.

Biography & Autobiography—Personal Memoirs • 6" x 9" • 384 pages • ISBN 978-0-593-65713-3 • $29.00 ($39.00 CAN)

NOT FOR SALE